REAL FIT

Kitchen

Fuel Your Body, Improve Energy, and Increase Strength with Every Meal

TARA MARDIGAN, R.D., AND KATE WEILER, C.H.C.

FAIR WINDS

To all the athletes who tirelessly put in the work, regardless of when you cross the finish line. You inspire us every day.

–Tara and Kate

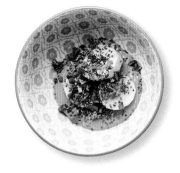

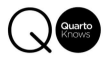

Quarto is the authority on a wide range of topics.

Quarto educates, entertains and enriches the lives of our readers—enthusiasts and lovers of hands-on living.

www.quartoknows.com

© 2015 Fair Winds Press

First published in the United States of America in 2015 by
Fair Winds Press, a member of
Quarto Publishing Group USA Inc.
100 Cummings Center
Suite 406-L
Beverly, Massachusetts 01915-6101
Telephone: (978) 282-9590
Fax: (978) 283-2742
quartoknows.com
Visit our blogs @quartoknows.com

19 18 17 16 15   1 2 3 4 5

ISBN: 978-1-59233-690-6

Digital edition published in 2015
eISBN: 978-1-62788-717-5

Library of Congress Cataloging-in-Publication Data

Mardigan, Tara.
    Real fit kitchen: ditch the protein powders, energy drinks, supplements, and more \with 100 simple homemade alternatives / Tara Mardigan, R.D. and Kate Weiler, C.H.C.—Digital ed.
            pages cm
    ISBN 978-1-59233-690-6
1. Cooking (Natural foods) 2. Functional foods. 3. Health.
I. Weiler, Kate. II. Title.
    TX741.M354 2015
    641.3'02—dc23
                              2015000599

Cover and book design by Laura McFadden Design, Inc.
Photography by Kristin Teig
Styling by Catrine Kelty

Printed and bound in China

The information in this book is for educational purposes only. It is not intended to replace the advice of a physician or medical practitioner. Please see your health care provider before beginning any new health program.

"I met Tara only months after I was diagnosed with celiac disease. At the time, I was competing in NCAA football at Harvard. Maintaining optimum nutrition in light of my newly diagnosed dietary restrictions was imperative. Today, as a professional athlete, I still reference several of the various nutritional concepts that Tara taught me."

—**Marco Iannuzzi**, professional athlete (Grey Cup champion wide receiver for the BC Lions of the Canadian Football League), investment advisor, speaker, philanthropist

"Kate's nutrition philosophy is exactly what our members were looking for. They knew the basics of nutrition, but Kate helped them take it to the next level with her integrative philosophy combined with the reality of life as an athlete. Our members couldn't say enough good things after sessions with her."

—**Joanna Roche**, spa director Westmoor Club, former director of Canyon Ranch, Lenox

"I can't recommend Kate more highly as a sports nutritionist. Kate completely dialed in to my struggles while training for the Boston Marathon. I was having GI distress and cramping during my runs, plus was bound to the couch feeling sick all day after every long run. After a couple of sessions with Kate, she eliminated all my issues and I have never felt more energy. I finished my first Boston Marathon at the age of 62 and beat my goal time."

—**Paul Lazar**, marathoner

"I learned way more from Kate in one session than I learned in five sessions with a top sports nutritionist!"

—**Breno Melo**, elite amateur Ironman triathlete

"After hearing Tara speak at the 2011 Boston Marathon Expo and deciding I needed to do something about my nutrition in order to improve my performance, I had a single consultation. The first 30 minutes were spent machine-gunning me with questions about what I ate, when I ate before exercise, and about my postworkout and race nutrition. Based on the information I gave her, she customized a nutrition plan for me which effected immediate benefits. In a couple of months, I dropped 15 pounds after making minor tweaks to my diet per Tara's recommendations. I cut an hour off of my Boston Marathon time because I was able to train smarter. She doesn't advocate dispensing with the guilty pleasures such as alcohol, coffee, or your favorite unhealthy foods; rather, she steers you toward the healthier choices available, which are just as fulfilling. After a consultation with Tara, I also became much more aware of selecting food based on how it is raised or grown. I would recommend her for improving elite or general athletic performance, losing weight, or just adopting a healthier lifestyle."

—**Mick Brown**, marathon and ultra-marathon runner

"I coach high school boys' and girls' swim teams and a master's swim team. Kate has helped elevate my swimmers' level of performance by teaching them how to properly fuel and hydrate themselves before, during, and after practice. Many of my swimmers were 'bonking' unknowingly due to lack of proper fuel and hydration and, therefore, not being able to swim to their potential. They no longer experience bonking during meets or during practice and have more energy and strength."

—**Jen Dutton**, high school swim and master's swim coach

"*Real Fit Kitchen* empowers the time-starved athlete to take control of their nutritional choices on the often-challenging and confusing road to wellness and high performance. It's like having your own personal sports nutritionists on call, whether you're a beginner or an elite athlete. This book provides a wealth of practical insight on what it takes to achieve and maintain a healthy lifestyle with easy-to-prepare, convenient recipes and accessible ingredients that do not disappoint on taste, bold flavors, or personality."

—**Larry Anderson**, head men's basketball coach, Massachusetts Institute of Technology

"As a professional athlete, I have to make sure that I am fueling my body with the right foods. The recipes found in *Real Fit Kitchen* are quick and easy for someone who is always on the go. If you're looking to increase your energy and improve your performance, this is the book for you."

—**Keith Wright**, professional basketball player, former Harvard Crimson basketball player

"Because of my nomadic lifestyle, eating healthy can be a challenge. *Real Fit Kitchen* is the nutrition bible for those always on the move. It's a blessing to learn how to make simple, nutritious meals—food that feeds the mind, body, and soul."

—**F. Stokes**, rapper and poet

"*Real Fit Kitchen* is a real find. No pills, powders, or potions—just delicious recipes to help keep you fit for life."

—**Ron Lawner**, former creative director and chairman of Arnold Worldwide

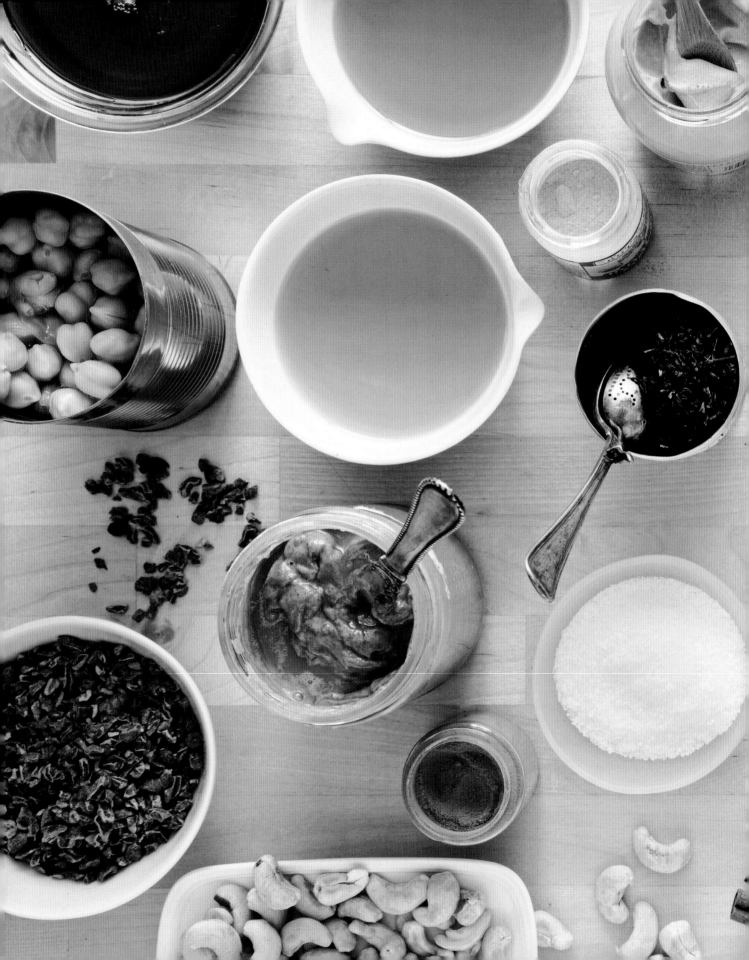

contents

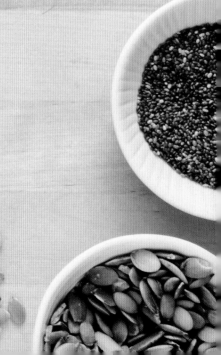

Preface

Tara: One of my earliest and favorite food memories is eating dinner with my older sister, Stacey. I was about five, she was eight. We were eating spaghetti at the dinner table before rushing off to gymnastics practice. My mom made a beautiful homemade red sauce with meatballs, but we were more interested in swirling the slippery pasta strands around our forks than in admiring her food.

We weren't interested in her red sauce or meatballs. We wanted our pasta smothered in butter and Parmesan cheese from that infamous green container. We even had a rule: If you couldn't see the cheese on the pasta because it had melted, you simply needed to add more "sprinkle cheese."

We filled our bellies with pasta, butter, and cheese as our mom shook her head that we were missing out on the best part—the part she made from scratch, with love and care. I didn't understand what she meant at the time. Food was food.

Gradually, I become more curious about the food on my plate. I was lucky. At home, we had fresh food, homemade lunches, and plenty of fruits and vegetables. We bought healthy ingredients. I still recall the smell of carob and spices at our local food co-op. Pizza was a treat. Sugared cereals were reserved for the occasional sleepover at a friend's house. And a meal at McDonald's was a highway stop on a long road trip (if everything else was closed). My mom's food was simple and healthy. I'm deeply appreciative of that now.

Growing up, I was a gymnast and noticed that food was a topic of interest in our group. Some girls were eating very little in an effort to stay slim. I'm not sure how I escaped this all-too-common fate, but I was more interested in how I could eat differently to be a better gymnast. What foods would give me more energy and power? From a very young age, I had sports nutrition on my radar.

As a registered dietitian, I try to help people connect with the basic concept that simple and healthy food will help them feel better and perform better. Trading convenience and processed foods for real, natural foods can have a lasting effect on day-to-day energy, mental focus, and muscle recovery (good-bye soreness), as well as of long-term health, wellness, and disease prevention. Getting people to ignore the lofty claims on modern products and believe that simple, pure food is best is, honestly, a tough sell.

I met Kate at the end of a long Boston winter in 2013. She was finishing her master's degree in nutrition at Northeastern University and was interested in the field of sports nutrition. She

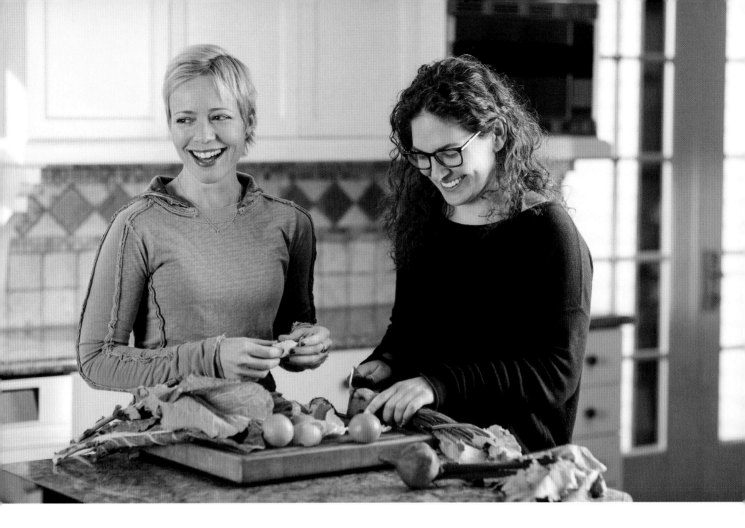

worked on a sports nutrition project with me for her final graduate school project. Kate's background as a high-level triathlete only validated my belief as to just how important real food is to performance. You don't get to compete at Kona, the world's most prestigious Ironman triathlon, by eating whatever you want.

Kate and I would meet once a week and talk nonstop about the maddening world of sports nutrition marketing. How can a product improve performance when it has corn syrup listed as the first ingredient and food coloring as the second? We'd just shake our heads at the many examples of brilliant marketing to athletes—essentially the brilliant marketing of *junk food*.

The conversation would always turn into a discussion about recipes or cooking. How did you make that bone broth? Have you ever made kombucha? How can you get wheatgrass to taste better? What's your favorite salt? Do you have a favorite sports drink or gel? What do you eat when you travel?

Those around us would listen to our unending food chatter and chuckle, "You two should write a cookbook for busy athletes."

So, we did just that. We hope the recipes in this book inspire you to choose natural ingredients, simple preparations, and a do-it-yourself attitude. Have fun, get messy, and when in doubt, put more color on the plate.

One last note: I still can't get enough buttered noodles with "sprinkle cheese."

—Tara A. Mardigan, M.S., M.P.H., R.D.
Nutritionist,
theplatecoach.com
@theplatecoach

Kate: I graduated from college and entered the world of information technology sales. To say it wasn't my thing is an understatement. I had always been interested in health and wellness and participated in athletics growing up, but never considered making a career of any of this. It was after my first Ironman triathlon that I realized that life was too short to wake up every day selling hardware and software.

I left my job and spent more time practicing yoga and reading books on nutrition. *In Defense of Food* by Michael Pollan changed my world. Understanding the food industry and how it impacts our education and our food recommendations made me mad and I wanted to do something about it. Brendan Brazier's book *Thrive* intrigued me. Why had I never even heard of many of these foods? I had been seeing a nationally acclaimed sports nutritionist to help me with my marathon running. Why hadn't she told me any of this? Why did I think a daily diet of pretzels, peanut butter, and sports drinks would prepare me properly for marathons? I realized that I needed to work in sports nutrition.

I'm not sure if it was pure luck or the universe saying that it was meant to be, but I sent Tara an email the week before I was supposed to start my internship for my master's degree asking if I could work with her. As Tara jokingly tells the story, she was dumbfounded that someone would have the audacity to email on such short notice, not realizing that she had students lined up years in advance to work with her. Hey, it never hurts to ask. Luckily, she made room for me to work with her and we clicked immediately.

When I realized the influence the food industry has on our eating recommendations, it inspired me to try to change that. The big food companies spend large amounts of money on product marketing, encouraging you to eat their product, but no one stands up for the food in the produce aisle because there isn't any money in that. My training partners and my clients were consuming products from big food companies because they thought these products were good for their bodies. They thought they were eating healthy, boosting their strength, and increasing their speed. Yet they were eating products that were only posing as health foods. So the question is, always, "What do I eat?"

The mission of this book is to help you eat real, delicious food. We want to introduce you to some wonderful ingredients, ones that you may not know about or may not know how to incorporate into your diet. We want to help you move away from products concocted by food scientists in a lab and empower you to create your own food: food that will give you more vitality and strength than you can imagine. For me, when I focused on eating real foods, my athletic performance soared. I was swimming, biking, and running faster than I had ever before. I was amazed by my clients' improvements, too. By making small, easy changes, they were breaking personal records and feeling phsically and mentally the best they had in years.

I owe a huge thank-you to my mother and my grandmother, who taught me that real food cooked at home is best. Growing up in a time of margarine and fat-free packaged foods, we always had real butter and homecooked meals made with a lot of love and attention. Looking back, I can now appreciate that the love that goes into the food can be just as nourishing as the nutrients that make up that food.

—Kate Weiler, M.S., C.H.C.
Sports Nutritionist
nutritionkate.com
@kkweiler

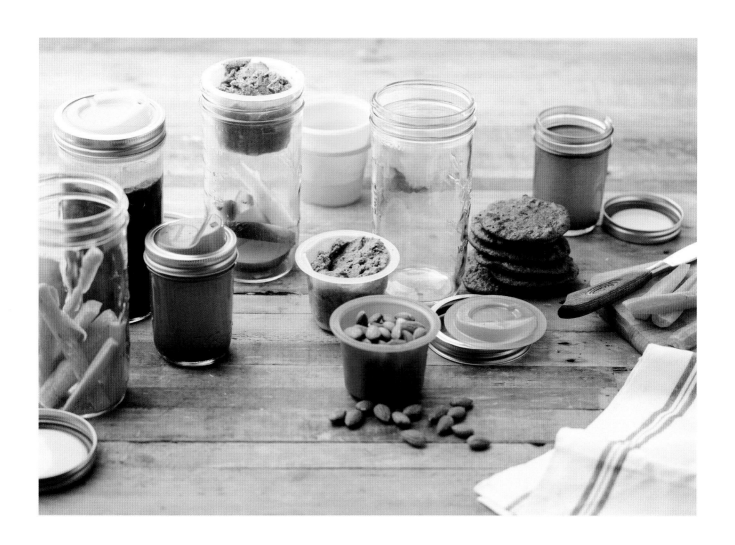

Introduction

We love food. We also love to sweat.

Our passion for food is connected to the way we move. There's nothing more satisfying than nourishing the body in a way that produces a steady, vibrant energy and a craving to be active each day. As nutritionists and athletes, we feel that a more streamlined food approach (not a nutrition approach) can do wonders to improve nutrition and overall well-being. It's simple, really; upgrading food choices on a consistent basis sets the stage for an active body and a calm mind.

Don't worry. Upgrading your food choices doesn't mean limiting your favorite foods or avoiding indulgences. That never works. We encourage a fresh outlook. Make your food simple, vibrant, wholesome, creative, and appealing. In a short time, the indulgences will be just that, occasional indulgences. Focus on eating what's good and you'll find you don't have as much interest in eating what's not as good.

Our recipes are easy to prepare and share with all ages. Each recipe is packed with nutrients that work for an athlete, a fit person, or a professional couch potato, all living under the same roof (although a side effect of this cookbook is greater fitness and less couch time). Our focus is on real ingredients, whole foods, and simple preparations. We're guessing that you don't have the time to be a top chef if you're pursuing other goals in life,

like working at a job you love, crushing your next road race, or fitting in a yoga class after a stressful workday. We want you to spend some quality time in the kitchen so you can be more efficient and energetic in your time outside the kitchen.

Often, especially for athletes, the emphasis is on numbers. Nailing the correct numbers. Calories. Fat. Sugar. Carbs. Ratios. We'd rather have you nail the ingredients. Be more competitive there. What's in your food? Make something from scratch using whole foods and it will be much easier to answer that question. Here's a choice: water with slices of fresh key lime in your favorite glass or lime-flavored hypersweet chemical-laden water in a plastic bottle with a flashy sugar-free, calorie-free label. We know which one we'd choose.

We want you to seek out and appreciate real food choices and forget about the numbers. That's our goal with this cookbook: real, vibrant, whole ingredients; a little more time in the kitchen; and a hefty dose of creativity. Welcome to *Real Fit Kitchen*.

REAL FOOD VS. PACKAGED FOODS

Many people are looking for a magic bullet that will increase speed, strength, weight loss, and energy. Sports nutrition companies are marketing packaged products and supplements for optimal fueling and recovery with ingredients that are supposed to catapult your performance to the next level. The problem is that most of these products further complicate foods that nature has already perfected, and food companies use their enormous assets to promote, not real food, but these packaged products and supplements.

The sports nutrition market is expected to grow over 80 percent by the year 2019. The market for supplements alone is a sizeable portion of that market. That means companies that can convince athletes of the performance benefits of their products are poised to make impressive profits. Some professional athletes sign multimillion-dollar sponsorship deals when they don't even use the products they are endorsing. In this crowded market, it is hard to know what to try, what to denounce as hype, and what can be downright counterproductive to health and performance.

Most of the sports nutrition advice emphasizes nutrients. How many calories should we eat? What percentage of carbohydrates, fat, and protein do we need? How many milligrams of vitamin C should we take? In our practices, we have found that most athletes do not focus on eating whole foods, which are naturally nutrient dense and filled with micronutrients and phytonutrients. We need to shift the focus to foods that are inherently packed with performance-optimizing benefits rather than ones created in chemistry labs.

We believe that food works synergistically, not in parts. Nutrients working together create more powerful health benefits than a synthetically created one taken alone does. Food created in nature does more good for the body than food created in a lab. This is why we stress eating whole eggs, not egg whites, eating citrus fruits and leafy greens rather than taking vitamin C supplements, and eating nuts instead of taking vitamin E supplements. Not only will you get a greater benefit and save money, you will not run the risk of detrimental side effects from unregulated and synthetic vitamins. Throughout the book, we point out some of the micronutrients and components so you can identify the benefits of certain foods. (In many cases, there are too many to list them all.) We can't say often enough: If you are eating whole food, you are on the right track.

Healthy eatery Hu Kitchen in New York City says, "It's not the omega-3 fatty acids in the salmon that make it healthy; it's the salmon in the salmon."

Most people look at a nutrition label for calories, protein, carbohydrates, and fat and overlook the ingredients list. Athletes focused on macronutrients often fail to be their own ingredient detectives and conventional sports nutrition doesn't emphasize reading the ingredient label. What is going to help you get stronger faster, recover more quickly, and perform your best has more to do with the ingredients than it does with the calories. Spend less time looking at the attention-grabbing claims on the front of the package and read the ingredient label on the back to decide if the ingredients are the best ones for you. You can eat the right amount of the right nutrients and consume what you think are perfect ratios, but still not find the success you are looking for because the low-quality food is sabotaging your diet. Eat less packaged food and more real food. Make an effort to know where your food comes from, buy local and organic—when possible—and you will see a huge difference in how you feel and perform.

OUR PHILOSOPHY, OUR RECIPES

Our recipes are packed with wholesome real foods to help you boost your performance. We look beyond the macronutrients of protein, fat, and carbohydrates and emphasize eating food naturally loaded with all the things that are going to help you reach your goals. By starting to incorporate more of these foods into your meals, you will:

- Increase energy and minimize fatigue.
- Recover faster between workouts.
- Be much more efficient and productive with workouts.
- Become stronger and faster.
- Strengthen your immune system.
- Lessen soreness and joint pain by quieting inflammation.
- Reach a healthy goal weight and improve body composition.

The world of nutrition today is confusing. There are scientific studies, the vast resources of large food companies, testimonials from athletes, the opinion of coaches, all with different viewpoints and voices.

So, what's really the best way to eat? There's only one answer to that question. You need to figure out what works best for you, and only you. There are common principles that support any healthy eating choice, but overall, there isn't one right way to eat for everybody, all the time. Things change; we like to call it "life creeping in."

Real Fit Values

Following are our ten principles that will work for everyone, no matter which eating pattern you choose to follow.

Paint your plate.

- **Plant based**—Make the majority of the foods you eat plant based. This is the number one thing you can do to improve your health and performance, and the health of the environment. Focus on eating fruits, vegetables, beans, nuts, seeds, grains, spices, and teas. Consume fewer animal foods and eat more plants.

- **Sustainable**—Think local, peak, seasonal, and small scale, whenever possible. The more you support local farmers, the more we'll be able to improve food quality as a community. Try to eat produce at the peak of its freshness. Look for farmer's markets, local farms, or local products highlighted on grocery shelves. A community garden or window box of fresh herbs—that's as local as you can get!

- **Strong**—Food should make you feel strong. If something makes you feel weak, tired, heavy, or sluggish, then it's not the best choice for you. Let food work for you.

- **Pure and Simple**—Eat food in its simplest form. Choose an orange, not a bottle of orange juice. Have plain whole yogurt, not a flavored, low calorie yogurt. The less processed a food is, the more of it you can have.

- **Colorful**—Paint your plate. It's that simple. Include as many vibrant colors as you can in each meal. If you tend to eat the same foods every day, try a different color combination. Make food grab your attention. It's your masterpiece. Let color guide you.

- **Consistent**—Set a realistic routine so you can be consistent with healthy behaviors. Create an approach simple enough that you can do it on a daily basis. That might require regular food shopping or prepping food the night before so you're ready for the next day.

- **Balanced**—Choose a variety of nutrients at each meal to help with portions, fullness, and overall nutrition balance. Too much protein? You're probably crowding out another nutrient. Too many fruits? You could be eating too much sugar. Choosing to eat different nutrient proportions relative to your activity level is a key to balanced eating. (More on this to come; see the Five Fingers method and Powerful Plates on pages 15 and 17).

- **Intuitive**—There are simple ways to make better food choices without being overly focused on the nuances and numbers of nutrition. Add a cup of frozen vegetables to a soup. Grab a banana at the breakfast staff meeting. Toss some beans into a salad. Drink more water during the workday. Split a dessert with a friend. The more seamless and intuitive your choices are, the better it is for you. Eating with intention and mindfulness helps guide more intuitive choices. Think out loud, "How can I make this better?" and you'll do just that.

- **Yours, Not Theirs**—The more you can cook, prepare, or flavor food yourself, the more control you have over what goes into it. Cook at home more often. When you're eating at a restaurant, ask for food the way *you* want it: vegetables roasted with olive oil and a lemon wedge, salad dressing on the side, or fresh fruit for dessert.

- **Real**—Change your perspective. Look at the ingredients not at the nutrition facts, percentages, health claims, and endorsements. Avoid artificial sweeteners and colors. Skip anything marketed as light/lite, low fat, low sugar, diabetic, or carb friendly. Real food requires no health claims.

We believe in balanced nutrition, not an all-or-nothing thinking. In our nutrition practices, the healthiest eaters are those who enjoy real food and respect it for its nourishment. They have active lifestyles but also realize the value of productive rest and relaxation.

Real food requires no health claims.

On any given day, the healthiest eaters will eat pretty darn well most of the time (80 percent) while also mindfully enjoying something downright indulgent some of the time (20 percent). A vivid vegetable-packed salad with quinoa, marinated tempeh, toasted pine nuts, and homemade cranberry dressing can be followed by a piece of spicy dark chocolate and a favorite glass of red wine.

Nothing is off limits. There are no cheat meals or cheat days, no being good or being bad. Avoid labeling yourself as being bad or cheating on your diet; food isn't a test. You are empowered to make decisions based on what suits your body and mind. No matter what we consume, our philosophy is that we are eating, not cheating. Good food choices fuel an active lifestyle on a sustainable level.

FIVE FINGERS: BALANCE

Focusing on the numbers of nutrition can detract from long-term sustainability. Sure, it can be helpful to keep track of intake and monitor progress, but not to the point where it's all consuming. Accountability, a solid support system, and motivation are important for making lifestyle changes that stay with us. Find the balance that allows you to monitor progress but let go of calorie counting, which is too specific a measurement to offer holistic progress.

We had the opportunity to meet award-winning food author, Michael Pollan, when he was at Harvard to talk about his book, *Cooked*. We shared that, as nutrition professionals, we were in total agreement that getting people to cook is the biggest way to improve nutrition and health and to strengthen relationships with friends and family. We also told him that we were intentionally leaving out nutrition facts for each recipe in this book. Our rationalization is simple: The recipes use only healthful and real ingredients, so there should be less focus on the numbers. He smiled in agreement and asked us to not get pressured into adding numbers that do not do justice to the true quality of the food.

Think 5: Every Nutrient, Every Meal

FIVE FINGERS: A BALANCED MEAL HAS ONE FROM EACH CATEGORY

❶ FRUITS/VEGETABLES (the more color, the better)	❷ CARBOHYDRATES	❸ PROTEINS	❹ HEALTHY FATS	❺ FLUIDS
fresh fruits	plain oatmeal, high-fiber/low-sugar cereal, gluten-free cereal	farm-fresh whole eggs	oils: extra-virgin olive, peanut, coconut, sesame, canola, avocado, ghee, grass-fed butter	water with lemon, lime, or cucumber slices for natural flavor
frozen fruits	fresh baked sourdough, sourdough spelt, 100% whole wheat bread, English muffins, pita sandwich thins, crackers, gluten-free bagels	fish, shellfish, poultry, grass-fed beef, bison, lamb, pork	avocado slices, guacamole, hummus	seltzer water, maple water, coconut water (avoid artificial sweeteners)
dried fruits (in small amounts)	high-fiber waffles or pancakes	beans, lentils, hummus, tofu, tempeh, edamame, soynuts	seeds: chia, hemp, sunflower, flax, sachi inchi, pumpkin	unsweetened tea: green, black, herbal (hot or iced), kombucha
fresh vegetables (nonstarchy)	brown rice, wild rice, whole wheat pasta, buckwheat (soba) noodles, gluten-free pasta	milk, yogurt, cottage cheese, cheese, kefir	unsweetened dried coconut, cacao nibs	fresh pressed juice diluted with water or seltzer
frozen vegetables (nonstarchy)	quinoa, couscous, bulgur, teff, farro, wheat berries, spelt, rye, millet, kamut, amaranth, barley, buckwheat	nuts, nut butters (peanut, almond, cashew, pistachio, soynut, macadamia, walnut)	nuts, nut butters (peanut, almond, cashew, pistachio, soynut, macadamia, walnut)	fresh pressed vegetable juice
fresh squeezed juice diluted with water or seltzer	starchy vegetables: potato, sweet potato, yam, turnip, winter squash, peas, corn, polenta, yucca, plantains, beets	protein powder: grass-fed whey, pea, hemp, egg white, chia, rice, sacha inchi, cricket, chlorella	omega-3 fish oil capsules, seaweed, vegan omega-3 capsules (microalgae oil)	milk: cow, goat, sheep, coconut, almond, rice, hemp, soy, lactose-free

THE FIVE FINGERS

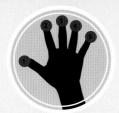

❶ Fruits/Vegetables

❷ Carbohydrates*†

❸ Proteins**

❹ Healthy Fats**

❺ Fluids

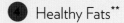
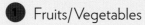
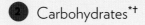

* Look for at least 4 grams of fiber per serving.   ** Some foods fall into multiple categories. For example, nuts and seeds contain both protein and fat.
† All starchy vegetables are considered carbohydrates.

We like visuals and use them with our clients. And we feel that eating with a balance of nutrient categories at each meal can help maintain energy, increase satisfaction, and supply the vitamins and minerals necessary for a healthy immune system. We encourage our clients to follow this chart to achieve balanced meals.

The Five Fingers method, (page 15), is a quick way to categorize nutrients and a visual way to remember each category.

Some foods fall into more than one category, and that's fine. Such a food can be a very efficient choice, as it offers you multiple nutrients. Nuts and fatty fish such as salmon or sardines are great examples; they have both protein and healthy fat. The Five Fingers chart helps you balance your meals so that you have one food choice from each category (or a few choices from each category for intense athletes). It's all about eating food from each category, at each meal.

Many athletes eat at least three protein choices at a meal but no fruits or vegetables or healthy fats. To balance the meal, limit yourself to one or two protein choices and add a fruit or vegetable and a healthy fat. Athletes doing intense exercise may have multiple choices but should still look to include foods from each category.

1. Fruits/Vegetables—The more the better, especially fresh fruits and vegetables locally grown. Think color for variety. We give our clients the green light with this category with these exceptions: juice, dried fruit, canned produce, and starchy vegetables, such as potatoes and corn.

2. Carbohydrates—Choose carbohydrates that are high in fiber. (Except when you are eating immediately before, during, or immediately after intense or prolonged exercise as the gut will not digest them in a timely manner. At those times, lower fiber carbohydrates are preferred.)

3. Proteins—Include protein from a variety of sources. People who choose animal proteins can also include a significant amount of plant-based proteins, too. Vegans and vegetarians should rely on whole food plant sources rather than on the more processed forms.

4. Healthy Fats—A little goes a long way with fat. Healthy fats help with satiety (fullness) and also improve the nutrient absorption of many antioxidant-rich fruits and vegetables. Fat can help both those trying to lose weight because it has appealing mouth feel and increases satisfaction, and, those trying to gain weight because it is calorie dense so it adds calories without a large increase in food volume.

5. Fluids—Hydration is so important. You should drink fluids with your meals and continuously throughout the day. Water and naturally flavored water are our favorite choices. Caffeine is fine in moderation and when consumed early in the day so it does not interfere with sleep.

the
PLATE
COACH

Powerful Plates

ENDURANCE

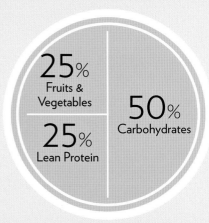

25% Fruits & Vegetables

25% Lean Protein

50% Carbohydrates

STRENGTH + ENDURANCE

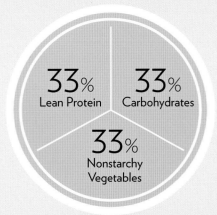

33% Lean Protein

33% Carbohydrates

33% Nonstarchy Vegetables

HEALTHY WEIGHT

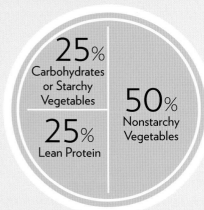

25% Carbohydrates or Starchy Vegetables

25% Lean Protein

50% Nonstarchy Vegetables

LESS ACTIVE

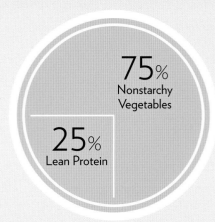

75% Nonstarchy Vegetables

25% Lean Protein

CHECKLIST

- ○ Slow your eating pace.
- ○ Use healthy fats for cooking and/or on top of vegetables/salad. A little goes a long way.
- ○ Hydrate with water. Keep it simple.
- ○ Flavor with spices, not excess salt.
- ○ Need to gain weight? Have another plate, and keep the same proportions.

- ○ Need to lose weight? Try a salad plate. Have nonstarchy vegetables, too.
- ○ Corn, peas, potato, plantains, and yucca count as carbohydrates not vegetables. They are starchy, so count them as such.
- ○ Choose high-fiber (at least 4 g per serving) carbohydrates, unless right before or right after intense exercise.

POWERFUL PLATES: CHOOSE YOUR PLATE BASED ON HOW YOU MOVE

We encourage our clients to take a simple visual approach when trying to figure out how much food to eat, *especially for the nighttime meal*, often the largest meal of the day. The plate visuals help guide you to arrange the food on your plate based on the type and level of activity you have participated in that day.

Finding the right amount of food to eat will change based on how active you are and the type of exercise you do. A marathon runner trying to gain muscle mass should be eating very differently than the CrossFit athlete who is unable to exercise due to a leg injury.

There are four Powerful Plates. Choose your plate, and keep in mind that it might be a different plate each day.

Trying to gain weight or lean muscle mass? Double (or triple) the plate but keep the proportions of nutrients the same. Use larger plates.

Trying to lose weight? Use salad plates. If you're still hungry, go for an extra plate or large bowl of nonstarchy vegetables with vinegar or lemon juice and spices to add flavor.

Endurance The Endurance Powerful Plate is designed for distance runners, cyclists, swimmers, cross-country skiers, triathletes, or any athlete doing continuous exercise for 2 or more hours in a day. This athlete requires more carbohydrates than others to best replenish muscle glycogen (the storage form of carbohydrates). If muscle glycogen isn't replenished, the athlete will struggle at the next workout session.

Strength and Endurance The Strength and Endurance Powerful Plate is designed for athletes in soccer, lacrosse, field hockey, tennis, basketball, gymnastics, golf, mixed martial arts, CrossFit, wrestling, vinyasa yoga, weight lifting, or any sport requiring both endurance and strength combinations. These sports generally include intense but intermittent bouts of exercise with brief rest periods mixed throughout the workout.

Healthy Weight The Healthy Weight Powerful Plate is designed for active people who work out for shorter durations (less than an hour) or with less intense exercise such as walking, water aerobics, or restorative/relaxing yoga.

Less Active The Less Active Powerful Plate is designed for minimal activity, due to injury or a hectic schedule. **The less active you are, the fewer carbohydrates you need**. Choose, instead, large amounts of nonstarchy vegetables. The Less Active Powerful Plate also works well at dinnertime for active people trying to lose weight, provided that high-fiber carbohydrates are included in earlier meals.

Upgrade Your Pantry

BASIC ITEMS AND INGREDIENTS TO HELP YOU MAKE THE MOST OF EVERY MEAL

Our kitchens are quite simple. You don't have to buy fancy kitchen tools or gadgets to make healthy food. But you'll want to start with some basic items and ingredients to help you make the most out of every meal.

One tool worth spending the money on is a high-performance blender with a plunger. It saves time, is easy to clean, and is less complicated to use than a food processer. You'll also want a **garlic press, citrus squeezer, citrus zester**, and a **whisk.**

Not all ingredients are created equal. The quality of the food is just as important as the food itself. An easy way to improve your health and overall well-being is to upgrade your staples. You want the best when buying items you use on a regular basis because you put them in your body every day. These ingredients should form the foundation of your meals:

Salt Try pink Himalayan sea salt or Celtic sea salt.

Cooking Oil and Fats Choose high-quality, expeller or cold-pressed, unrefined and unfiltered fats and oils: animal fats from grass fed animals and high-quality plant oils. We like extra-virgin olive oil, coconut oil (especially at higher heat), high-quality expeller-pressed organic canola oil (also known as rapeseed oil), pumpkin seed oil, hemp oil, and avocado oil. Flaxseed oil, rich in omega-3 fatty acids, can be used as a noncooking oil.

Butter Buy butter that comes from grass-fed cows raised without hormones and antibiotics. Ghee is a type of clarified butter that lacks casein, a digestive irritant for some.

Spices Check the ingredients and avoid additives, preservatives like citric acid, anti-caking agents, sulfites, or even sugar.

Sweeteners We like pure maple syrup and raw honey and buy local products.

Nut Butter Use natural nut butters—ones where the only ingredient on the label is nuts.

Bread Buy bread from a local artisanal bakery. We love sourdough—which is fermented and contains probiotics and enzymes—sprouted bread, or a good millet bread.

Eggs Find local, pasture-raised eggs. If you can't find local eggs, choose eggs from organically raised, free-range chickens that have not been fed antibiotics or hormones.

Condiments Check ingredient labels to avoid hidden sugars, preservatives, and unnecessary fillers.

Protein Powder We are big fans of getting protein from real food. But protein powder may have its benefits for busy athletes. We recommend hemp protein, brown rice protein, pea protein, or a minimally processed grass-fed whey protein. Plant-based protein powder blends are also available.

Milk, Cheese, and Yogurt Always choose the best quality milk, cheese, and yogurt you can find, ideally from local sources. Choose grass-fed dairy from free ranging cows.

TARA AND KATE'S TOP TWENTY

We love to buy what is fresh and local to eat seasonally. Food in season and local hasn't traveled far and retains more nutrients. When grocery shopping, we pay attention to foods that are most vibrant and are calling our names. We have favorite foods, our go-to ingredients, that are always in our kitchen.

1. Greens. Whether it's spinach, kale, arugula, collards, or bok choy, we always keep greens on hand for their high level of nutrients, fiber, and anti-inflammatory benefits.

2. Eggs. Local neighborhood eggs taste better and are better for you. The yolks are a rich deep orange/yellow hue and they are often larger than conventional eggs. They provide both protein and lutein.

3. Extra-virgin olive oil. High-quality olive oil is heart-healthy and satiating. We use expensive high-quality olive oil for dressings and dips.

4. Chia seeds and hemp seeds. Chia seeds and hemp seeds are packed with nutrients. We love their energy-boosting and anti-inflammatory properties. We add them to smoothies, yogurt, salads, nut butter, and pudding to boost their nutrition benefits.

5. Cacao nibs. Nibs, the raw, natural source of chocolate, are packed with antioxidants, mood-elevating phytonutrients, and the minerals magnesium, iron, and calcium. A spoonful to a smoothie, bowl of yogurt, cereal, or pudding goes a long way.

6. Spice blends. We rely on spice blends to add flavor to vegetables, proteins, and grains without adding extra fat or salt. Spices provide immune-supporting phytonutrients. Experiment with various blends such as Baharat and Ras el Hanout.

7. Apple cider vinegar. We use organic, raw, unfiltered, and unpasteurized apple cider vinegar, which is a bit cloudy. It's a rich source of probiotics and may help with digestion and immune health. Diluted with water, it may help control blood sugar as it blocks some the digestion of starchy foods. Processed versions do not have the same health benefits.

8. Nut or seed butter. It is a fast, inexpensive, accessible food that is an efficient balance of protein, healthy fats, fiber, vitamins, and minerals. When buying a commercial version instead of homemade, check the ingredients—look for nuts or seeds with a little salt (and no fillers).

9. Turmeric. A member of the ginger family, turmeric is a powerful anti-inflammatory that also has anticancer benefits. It can be used to flavor soups, vegetables, and dressings. If you find turmeric too bitter, try adding a few drops of honey.

10. Bananas. This potassium-packed, low-to medium-glycemic fruit is portable, cheap, and accessible. Use bananas past their peak for smoothies or for baking. Or peel, slice, and freeze overripe ones and add them to recipes for an ice cream–like texture.

11. Pumpkin seeds. Also known as pepitas, these seeds provide a powerful mixture of antioxidants, minerals, healthy fat, fiber, and protein. Raw or roasted, shelled or unshelled, pumpkin seeds can be added to salads, shakes, trail mix, or sprinkled on top of a sweet potato.

12. Chickpeas and lentils. Canned chickpeas (a.k.a. garbanzo beans) are inexpensive, have a long shelf life, and are easy to add to salads or soups. We toss chickpeas into the blender with olive oil and spices for a speedy homemade hummus. The fiber and protein help with satiety and portion control.

13. Tea. Green tea, especially the Japanese varieties (sencha, gyokuro, and matcha) is rich in polyphenols known as EGCG, a strong antioxidant. Black and oolong teas found in more popular tea blends are less effective because the tea leaves have been processed and fermented, destroying some of the polyphenol content. Steep green tea for 8 to 10 minutes to optimize the polyphenol benefit and drink within an hour.

14. Edamame. These young soybeans in the pod provide a whole food, plant-based protein that's rich in isoflavones. Soy in highly processed powder and pill form can be problematic for health; but whole forms of soy such as edamame, tofu, soy nuts, and tempeh are good for you. Keep frozen edamame, shelled or unshelled, on hand.

15. Maca powder. Maca, a plant native to the Peruvian Andes has been used to increase strength and energy for thousands of years. Available in powder form, maca contains minerals, phytonutrients, and plant sterols thought to help block cholesterol absorption in the blood. It adds a nutty and slightly sweet flavor to drinks, smoothies, soups, proteins, and desserts.

16. Cinnamon. Cinnamon may help balance blood sugar levels and has antibacterial and anti-fungal properties. Use it to add a sweet flavor and rely less on larger amounts of sugar from maple syrup or honey. Cinnamon has a strong taste so try it in small amounts to start. We also use cinnamon sticks in tea or in hot water.

17. Sea salt. Using a high-quality sea salt, in either chunky crystals or flakes, adds trace minerals, including potassium, iodine, magnesium, and calcium, as well as sodium. Pink Himalayan, Persian Blue, and Celtic are good choices.

18. Maple syrup. Pure maple syrup has antioxidants and minerals and is less processed than white sugar, which is why we use it more often than other sugars when cooking. That said, it's still sugar and should be used in small amounts. As sappy as it sounds, we are New Englanders, and we love the "taste of the tree."

19. Mustard. Mustard is a versatile condiment. We keep it in multiple forms; yellow mustard, French-style Dijon mustard, mustard seeds, and mustard powder. Mix a spoonful of mustard into a homemade salad dressing or marinade. Mustard just makes everything better. Toast mustard seeds in a skillet and add to a sandwich, salad, sides, or an entree.

20. Salmon and sardines. The anti-inflammatory omega-3 fatty acids found in all fatty fish are good for you, but it's best to eat the smallest fish because they contain fewer environmental toxins such as PCBs (polychlorinated biphenyls), and mercury. Look for fresh or brands canned in olive oil, not sunflower oil, preferably with the bones.

How to Use This Book

We left out calories and nutrition numbers on our recipes on purpose. Sitting down to a meal should be a pleasurable event, not one where you are stressed or anxious or caught up in numbers. If you focus on eating good whole food, you will nourish your body and optimize your health and athletic performance much more than you would by taking out a scale, calculator, or calorie-counting app.

Instead of numbers, we provide each of our recipes with nutrition tags.

The first tag pertains to timing: the best time to eat in relation to your workout **Preworkout, Postworkout, Nutrient-Packed Mainstays,** or **Nutrient-Packed Treats**.

Preworkout—These recipes are higher in carbohydrates to provide muscle and mental energy. The foods are easy to digest and are appropriate to eat two hours or less before exercise and activity.

Postworkout—These recipes combine easy-to-digest carbohydrates and a protein to help with glycogen replenishment and muscle recovery and to prepare the body for its next workout. Recovery nutrition has been dominated by the notion that a precise 4:1 ratio of carbohydrates to protein is ideal. This has opened the door for food companies to produce heavily processed products that precisely fit this ratio and is the optimal way for the body to recover. Actually, many of these products contain inflammatory ingredients that may be inhibit recovery, not help it. Our post-workout recipes may not always fit the precise 4:1 ratio, but real food combinations are the best way to fuel the body.

Nutrient-Packed Mainstay—These recipes include fiber, healthy fat, and protein and are very nutrient dense. They are reliable go-to choices that are balanced, sustaining, immune supportive, and will help decrease inflammation. Because they are packed with slow-to-digest nutrients, these recipes are best eaten when you have at least 2 hours to digest the food before exercise.

Nutrient-Packed Treat—These recipes are for desserts or treats that are packed with more nutrients than your typical indulgence. Though they are much healthier versions of traditional desserts and candy, they should still be viewed as treats.

"A recipe has no soul. You, as the cook, must bring soul to the recipe."

—Thomas Keller, American chef, restaurateur, and cookbook writer

The second set of tags is based on the recipe's characteristics. These include **Gluten Free, Dairy Free, Vegan,** and **Low FODMAP.**

Gluten Free—Excludes gluten, a protein found in wheat and related grains, including barley and rye.

Dairy Free—Excludes milk and milk products from animals such as cows, sheep, and goats.

Vegan—Excludes all animal products.

Low FODMAP—Limits FODMAPs. The initialism FODMAP is derived from Fermentable, Oligo-, Di-, Monosaccharides, and Polyols. FODMAPs are types of carbohydrates including fructans, galactans, polyols, fructose, and lactose. They draw water into the intestinal tract and may not be digested or absorbed well if eaten in excess. This allows bacteria to ferment and may cause gas and bloating. The restriction of FODMAPs in the diet has been found to have a beneficial effect for sufferers of irritable bowel syndrome, colitis, and other functional gastrointestinal disorders. For more information on FODMAPs, go to katescarlata.com. Kate is a digestive health expert working in the area of FODMAPs.

The mission of *Real Fit Kitchen* is to help you eat real, delicious food. We want to expose you to some wonderful ingredients—some you may not know about, some you may not know how to incorporate into your meals. We want to help you move away from products concocted by food scientists in a lab and empower you to create your own food—food that will give you more vitality and strength than you can imagine.

We give you full permission to make changes to the recipes. If you do not like an ingredient or cannot find an ingredient in a recipe, feel free to take it out or substitute something else. Buy what is in season and add it to the recipes. Be creative in the kitchen. Don't be afraid to make mistakes. Have fun, and make the recipes your own.

PART I

Food Swaps

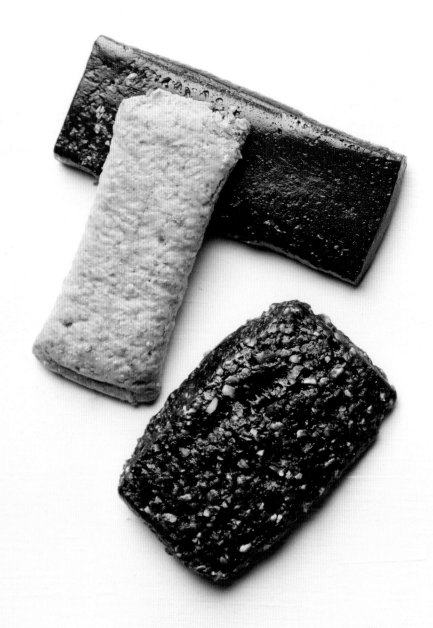

"Goodbye to energy bars."

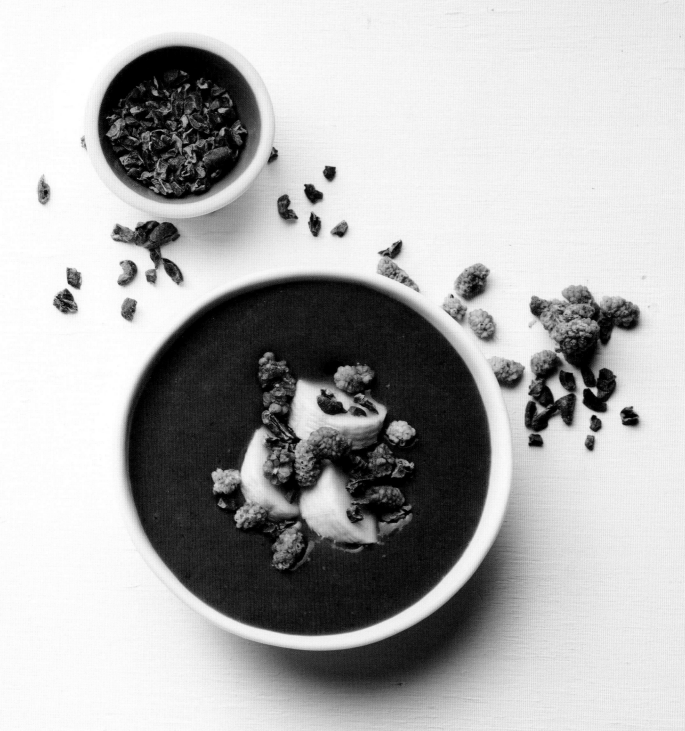

"Hello to Kate's Kona Bowl!"

CHAPTER 1

Breakfast

"Breakfast is the most important meal of the day." We've heard that often but it's true only if you fill your breakfast plate with nutrient-rich foods that will give you long-lasting energy, not with conventional breakfast foods that are full of sugar, salt, and fat. In this chapter, we offer you our favorite power breakfast ideas, foods that will motivate you and give you enough energy for a killer workout—but feel free to eat these foods any time of the day!

Fingertip Frittatas

Kale and Lox Scramble

Sunrise Plantains

Powerhouse Pancakes

Speedcakes

Egg McMardigans

Halloumi with Fig and Avocado

Kate's Kona Bowl

Cocoa Power Porridge

Crunchy Buckwheat Granola

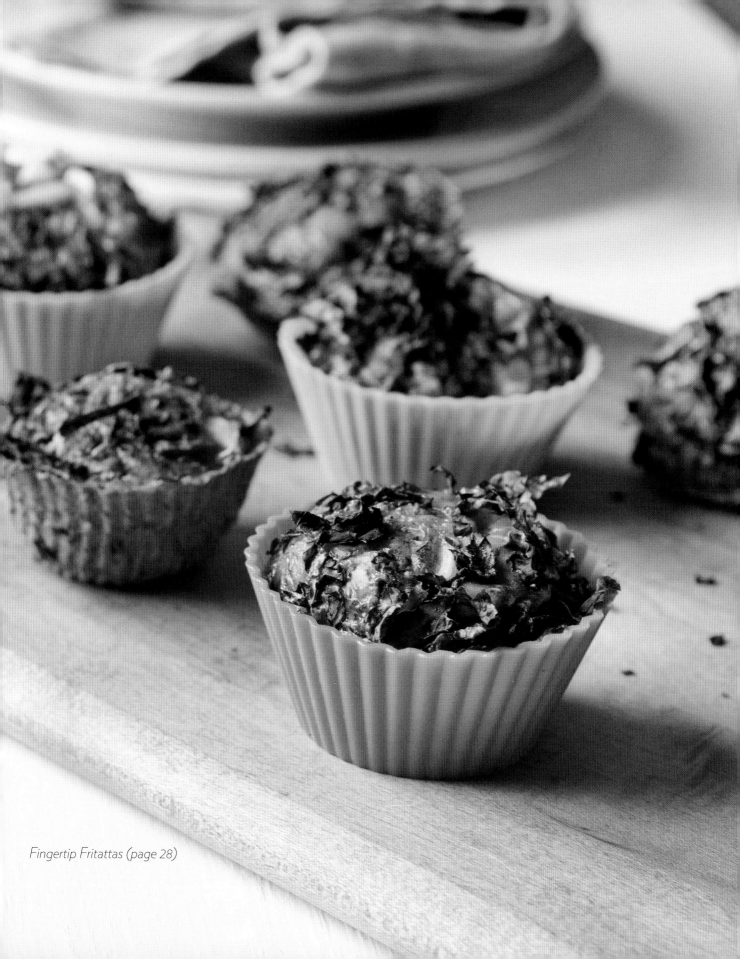

Fingertip Fritattas (page 28)

Fingertip Fritattas

When you're busy, it's easy to pick up packaged foods or buy a muffin at a coffee shop after a run. Instead, try our quick and easy frittatas, a portable version of eggs and vegetables. You can make these ahead of time, keep them in the refrigerator, and grab one as you are running out the door.

2 tablespoons (18 g) coconut oil or grass-fed butter

11 organic pasture-raised eggs

1 teaspoon turmeric

1 teaspoon cayenne pepper

2 teaspoons (12 g) sea salt

2 teaspoons (4 g) black pepper

1 cup (67 g) kale, chopped

¼ cup (40 g) onion, chopped

Preheat the oven to 350°F (180°C) and liberally grease the muffin tin with coconut oil.

Wisk together the eggs, turmeric, cayenne, salt, and pepper.

Combine the kale and onions in a separate bowl.

Fill muffin cups three-quarters full with the egg mixture.

Spoon kale and onions into each muffin cup.

Bake for 20 minutes.

Servings: About 4

Notes: Try adding other vegetables like red peppers or baked sweet potato chunks to the frittatas.

DID YOU KNOW? Eggs have been vilified as unhealthy due to the amount of cholesterol they contain. Recent studies have shown that this cholesterol has a fairly small effect on the body's blood-level cholesterol, less than previously thought. So, yes, you can and should eat the whole egg rather than just the egg whites. The yolks provide omega-3 fatty acids, vitamin E, vitamin B5, vitamin A, vitamin D, and lutein and choline. Organic eggs from pasture-fed chickens may be more expensive, but they are worth it because they have higher nutrient levels than eggs laid by caged hens.

▶ POSTWORKOUT ▶ NUTRIENT-PACKED MAINSTAY ▶ GLUTEN FREE ▶ DAIRY FREE

Kale and Lox Scramble

This is one of our favorite go-to meals after a long morning of training because it's fast, easy to make, and bursting with protein, omega-3 fatty acids, and antioxidants that aid in muscle recovery. Add a pinch of turmeric, which has anti-inflammatory properties, and you'll have one exceptional breakfast. Modify the recipe to suit your tastes by adding vegetables you have on hand like carrots, zucchini, or peppers.

1 teaspoon coconut oil, grass-fed butter or grass-fed ghee

½ cup (77 g) chopped onion

1½ cup (100 g) chopped kale, collard greens, or swiss chard

4 ounces (120 g) wild smoked salmon

4 eggs

Sea salt, black pepper, and turmeric to taste

Heat the coconut oil or butter on medium heat in a medium-size pan.

Sauté the onions and kale (or other leafy greens) for 3 minutes.

Add the smoked salmon and sauté for 1 minute.

Crack the eggs right in the pan and immediately stir with a spatula. Scramble the eggs, salmon, kale, and onions together.

Sprinkle with salt, pepper, and turmeric (optional) to taste.

Servings: 2

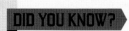 **DID YOU KNOW?** Salmon is rich in omega-3, a fatty acid that may help with joint health.

▶ POSTWORKOUT ▶ NUTRIENT-PACKED MAINSTAY ▶ GLUTEN FREE ▶ DAIRY FREE

Sunrise Plantains

We love plantains for their energy-boosting and blood sugar-stabilizing properties. Serve these plantains—which look like a bright, bold sun—with eggs for a perfect breakfast, or take them with you for a portable snack.

1 large plantain, sliced into ¼ -inch (6 mm) coins

1 teaspoon coconut oil

1 teaspoon pure maple syrup

½ teaspoon Hungarian paprika

¼ teaspoon cinnamon

¼ teaspoon sea salt

1 teaspoon olive oil or garlic-infused olive oil

Heat a pan on medium-high heat and add the coconut oil.

Mix the spices together in a bowl with the extra-virgin olive oil. Coat the plantains with this mixture by massaging it in with your hands, covering the plantains as evenly as possible.

Cook for 5 to 8 minutes on each side.

Servings: 2

Notes: *You can find plantains at most large grocery stores with an international foods section or at smaller Caribbean and Latin markets. Like bananas, the greener ones are less ripe and more starchy. Allow them to ripen, turn yellow with a few black spots, and they will be sweeter.*

DID YOU KNOW? **Plantains, a staple in Caribbean cooking, are large, green bananas that require cooking (boiled, fried, grilled, or roasted) before eating. A cup of plantains will give your body potassium, fiber, vitamin A, vitamin B6, and magnesium.**

▶ PREWORKOUT ▶ NUTRIENT-PACKED MAINSTAY ▶ GLUTEN FREE ▶ VEGAN ▶ DAIRY FREE
▶ LOW FODMAP

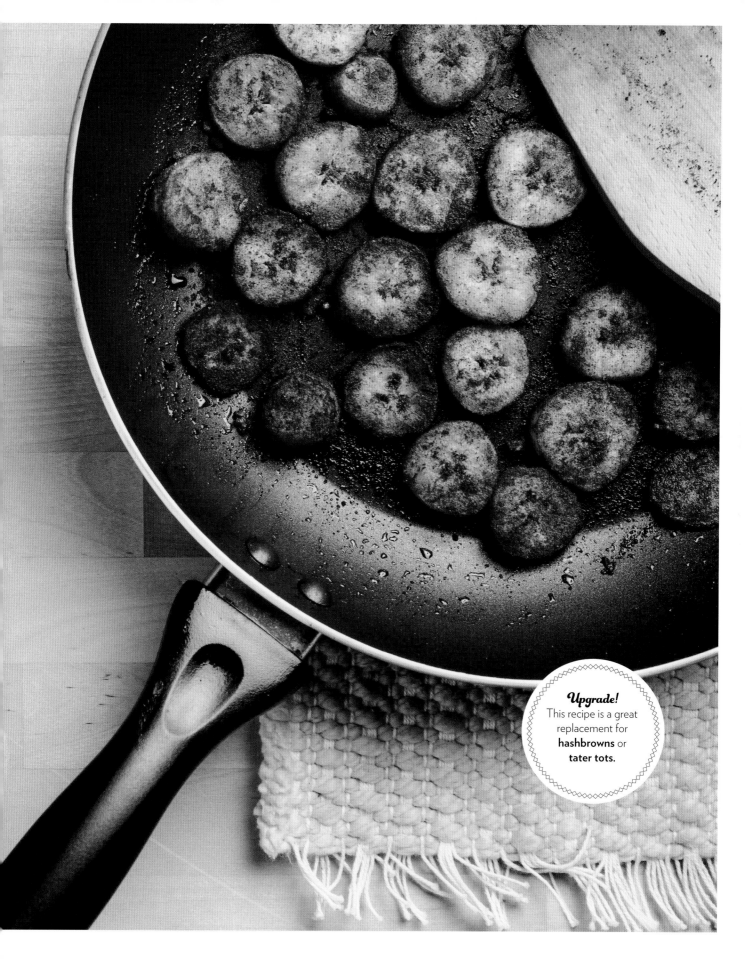

Upgrade!
This recipe is a great replacement for **hashbrowns** or **tater tots.**

Powerhouse Pancakes

Pancakes are a great way to quality-carb up before a race but most pancakes lack nutrients and are hard to digest, leaving you feeling lethargic and bloated. These pancakes are made with healthy, easy-to-digest ingredients that will help you compete like a pro. Top with pure maple syrup and enjoy!

- 1 cup (128 g) millet flour
- ½ teaspoon baking soda
- 2 teaspoons (9 g) baking powder
- 2 eggs
- ½ cup (122 g) baked sweet potato or canned sweet potato
- 1 cup almond (234 ml) milk or rice milk
- 1 teaspoon coconut oil, grass-fed butter, or grass-fed ghee
- 1 tablespoon (20 g) pure maple syrup

Combine all the dry ingredients in a mixing bowl.

In another bowl, wisk together the eggs, sweet potato, and almond milk.

Combine wet and dry ingredients and mix thoroughly.

Heat coconut oil or butter on medium heat.

Scoop about one-sixth of the batter for each pancake and cook for 2 minutes. Turn the pancakes over and cook for 1 minute.

Servings: 6

Upgrade!
This recipe is a great replacement for any carb-heavy breakfast food like **regular pancakes, bagels,** or **muffins.**

DID YOU KNOW? **Sweet potatoes provide long-lasting energy. Easy to digest and full of the antioxidant beta-carotene and vitamin C, sweet potatoes are one of our favorite powerhouse foods.**

▶ PREWORKOUT ▶ NUTRIENT-PACKED MAINSTAY ▶ GLUTEN FREE ▶ DAIRY FREE
▶ LOW FODMAP

Speedcakes

These pancakes are simple to make from ingredients we stock regularly in our kitchen. They are great to eat before or after a workout. Make them ahead of time, spread with nut butter and fold in half, and you have a portable pancake sandwich.

2 medium bananas

4 organic pasture-raised eggs

2 tablespoons (22 g) chia seeds

1 teaspoon cinnamon

½ teaspoon sea salt

1½ teaspoons vanilla

1 tablespoon (14 g) coconut oil, ghee, or grass-fed butter for cooking

Chopped nuts, fruit, or pure maple syrup for topping (optional)

In a blender, combine the bananas, eggs, chia seeds, cinnamon, salt, and vanilla.

Heat the coconut oil or butter in a large pan over medium-high heat.

Use a ½-cup (115 g) measure to scoop the batter into the pan.

Cook the pancakes for about 1 minute, until bubbles appear, then flip them and cook for another minute.

Add more oil to the pan, if necessary, as you continue to make the remaining pancakes.

Servings: 4 small pancakes

Upgrade!
This recipe is a great replacement for **traditional pancakes** or **bagels**.

▶ PREWORKOUT ▶ POSTWORKOUT ▶ GLUTEN FREE ▶ DAIRY FREE ▶ LOW FODMAP

Egg McMardigans

When Tara was very young, her father, a basketball coach for thirty years, told her that he invented Egg McMardigans and that Mickey D's simply borrowed it from him. Tara still believes this is true!

3 eggs

1 tablespoon (15 ml) olive oil

2 tablespoons (18 g) pine nuts

1 roasted red pepper, chopped and drained

2 cups (100 g) arugula or spinach

½ teaspoon sea salt

½ teaspoon black pepper

2 gluten-free English muffins (or your favorite bread)

1 tablespoon grass-fed butter (optional)

Add the oil to the pan and heat on low-medium heat.

Add the eggs, then the pine nuts and roasted red pepper on top (or to the side if using a larger pan). Salt and pepper to taste. Cook for about 2 to 3 minutes, then add the greens. Cook for another 2 to 3 minutes or until the yolks are the desired firmness and the greens just begin to wilt.

Serve the eggs on your favorite English muffin, bread, or toast.

Servings: 2

Notes: Tara swears by lemon-infused olive oil for this recipe. Add mini colorful sweet bell peppers that take just a minute to chop, and try scrambling the eggs.

▶ PREWORKOUT ▶ POSTWORKOUT ▶ NUTRIENT-PACKED MAINSTAY ▶ GLUTEN FREE ▶ DAIRY FREE ▶ LOW FODMAP

Halloumi with Fig and Avocado

Halloumi, a firm and salty cheese made from a combination of goat and sheep milk, is the perfect vehicle for a variety of flavors. In this recipe, puréed fig and avocado slices combine for a carbohydrate/protein/healthy fat combination that is a balanced and nourishing breakfast or snack.

6 to 8 fresh figs, stems cut off and quartered

1 ripe avocado

Juice of 1 small lime

1 tablespoon (14 g) coconut oil

1 package (8 ounces, or 225 g) halloumi cheese, cut into 8 slices

Black pepper to taste

Purée the chopped figs in a food processor or blender. Place them in a small bowl.

Slice the avocado into 8 thin slices and cover them with the lime juice.

Heat the coconut oil in the pan and add the halloumi slices. Cook for 2 to 3 minutes on each side until a dark crust forms. Remove the cheese.

Spread each cheese slice with a spoonful of the fig purée and top with an avocado slice.

Serve immediately. This tastes best when the cheese is still warm.

Notes: *This recipe can be made without the avocado, but pairing the salty cheese with the fig purée is a must. For a twist, grill the halloumi on skewers.*

▶ POSTWORKOUT ▶ NUTRIENT-PACKED MAINSTAY ▶ GLUTEN FREE

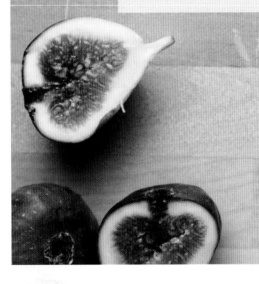

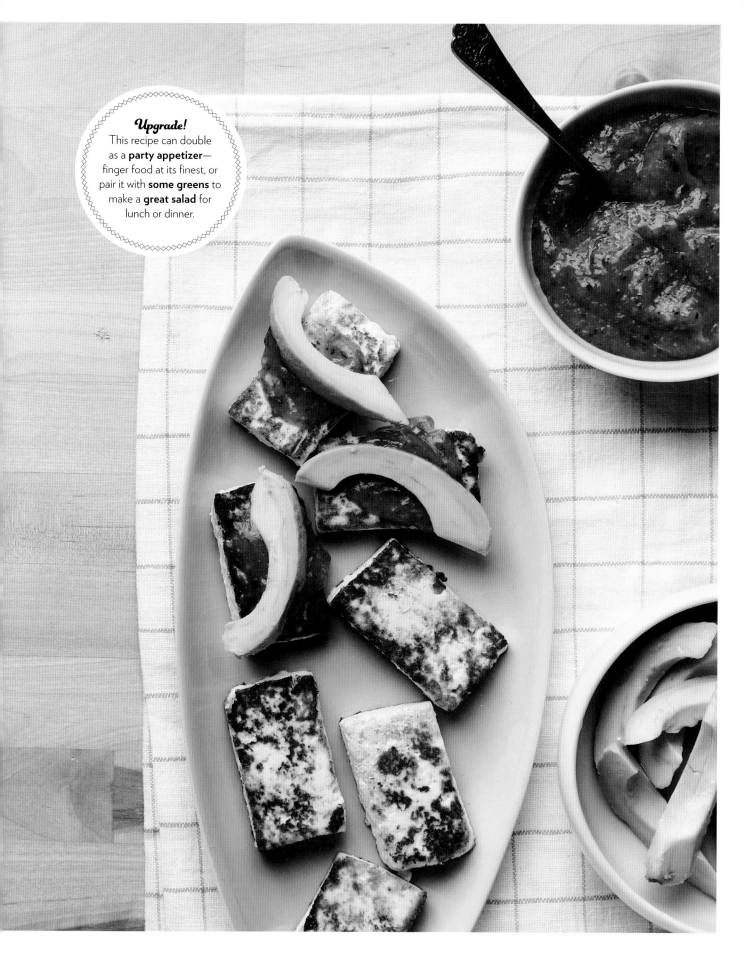

Upgrade!
This recipe can double as a **party appetizer**—finger food at its finest, or pair it with **some greens** to make a **great salad** for lunch or dinner.

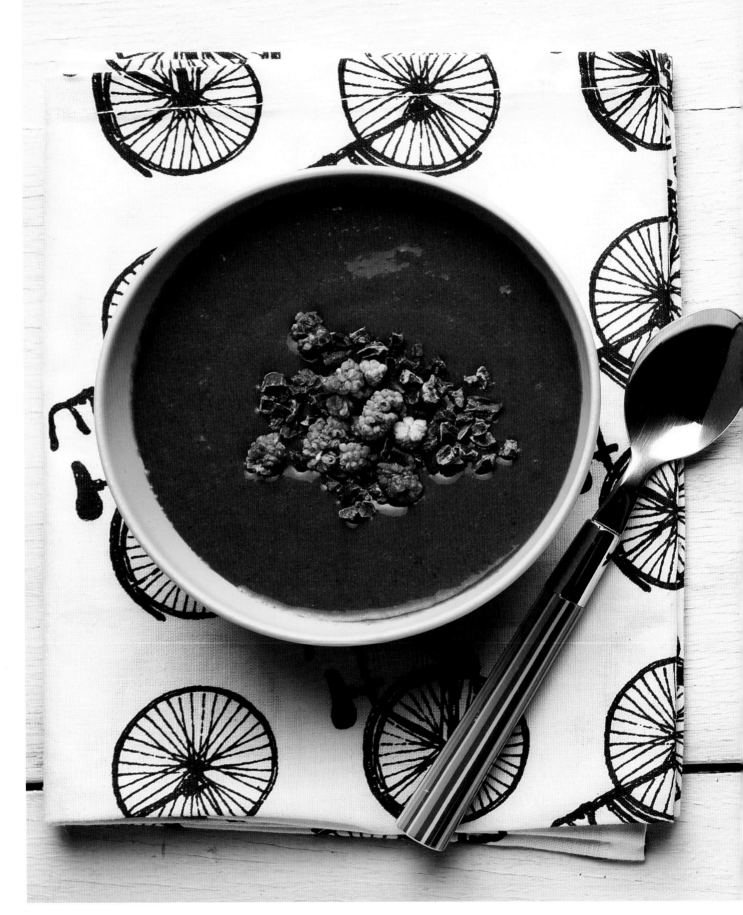

Kate's Kona Bowl

In Kona, Hawaii, there is a little hut on Ali'i Drive where professional and amateur Ironman triathletes alike line up for the one menu item: açaí bowls. When Kate was there to compete in the Ironman, she couldn't get enough of these bowls, and when she came back home, she tried to re-create them in her kitchen. Nothing seemed to match those açaí bowls in Kona. Kate came across the site Breakfast Criminals and convinced Ksenia, the founder, to share one of her recipes. Check out her website at www.breakfastcriminals.com.

3½ ounces (100 g) frozen açaí (or look for a frozen packet or pouch)

1 banana

½ cup (125 g) frozen strawberries

½ cup (90 g) frozen mango

⅔ cup (160 ml) coconut water or maple water

¼ cup (60 ml) unsweetened aloe vera juice

1 teaspoon maca powder

For topping:

1 tablespoon raw cacao nibs

1 tablespoon mulberries (optional)

Combine all the ingredients in a blender.

If the mixture is too thick, slowly add almond milk or water and blend until smooth.

Servings: 1

Note: *Get creative with toppings! Try adding berries, sliced banana, unsweetened coconut flakes, goji berries, sliced almonds, or chia seeds.*

Ugrade!
This recipe is a great replacement for **cold cereal** or **oatmeal** at breakfast or for **sorbet** or **other dessert.**

DID YOU KNOW? Açaí berries are known for their high level of antioxidants, chemicals that help keep you healthy by blocking free radicals that can damage cells.

▶ PREWORKOUT ▶ POSTWORKOUT ▶ GLUTEN FREE ▶ DAIRY FREE ▶ VEGAN
*Low FODMAP-friendly: Use frozen pineapple chunks instead of mango.

Cocoa Power Porridge

Amaranth is a nutrient-dense grain that is easy to digest, making it a great way to quality-carb up before a race or to eat for breakfast after a morning workout. Kate often eats this porridge the day before Ironman races to prepare her muscles.

½ cup (97 g) amaranth

1¼ (294 ml) cups water

¼ teaspoon sea salt

1 teaspoon maca powder

2 tablespoons (11 g) cacao powder

1 tablespoon (20 g) pure maple syrup

1 banana, sliced

Combine the amaranth and water in a saucepan. Bring to a boil, then reduce to a simmer. Cover and simmer on low for 15 minutes, stirring occasionally.

Stir in sea salt, maca, cacao powder, and maple syrup.

Serve topped with sliced banana.

Servings: 2

DID YOU KNOW? Amaranth is high in protein and a good source of the amino acids lysine and methionine, which are found in only small amounts in other grains. It contains four times the calcium and twice the iron and magnesium as wheat. Maca can help your body handle cortisol, a hormone that is linked to stress.

❯ PREWORKOUT ❯ POSTWORKOUT ❯ NUTRIENT-PACKED MAINSTAY ❯ GLUTEN FREE ❯ DAIRY FREE ❯ VEGAN ❯ LOW FODMAP

Crunchy Buckwheat Granola

We love granola! We eat it for breakfast and bring it as a portable snack when we travel to races. This recipe is easy to make ahead of time and can be doubled to make more. We also like to add it to our Cashew Chia Concoction (page 67). Many store-bought granolas have hidden ingredients and more sugar than a candy bar—not exactly what we consider healthy.

2 cups (240 g) buckwheat groats

½ cup (75 g) raisins or dried cherries (or a mixture)

½ cup (32 g) pepitas

2 tablespoons (11 g) raw cacao powder

1 teaspoon maca powder

2 tablespoons (40 g) pure maple syrup

1 teaspoon sea salt

Set the oven to its lowest setting or the dehydrator mode.

Rinse the buckwheat under cold water.

Combine all the ingredients in a bowl and stir them together.

Spread the granola mixture in a thin layer on a baking sheet and place in the oven for 1 hour.

Remove from the oven, let it cool, and store it in an airtight container to keep fresh longer.

Servings: 4

Notes: You can soak buckwheat in a bowl of cold water for 6 to 8 hours to sprout the grain. This will activate enzymes and provide more nutrients. It's not necessary, but with some planning, it's easy to do.

Upgrade!
Served with milk for a traditional granola or with warm milk for a porridge, this recipe is a great replacement for **cereal** or **store-bought granola.**

DID YOU KNOW? Despite its name, buckwheat is not related to wheat and is a pseudograin in the same family as rhubarb and sorrel. Easier for most people to digest than other whole grains, buckwheat has been shown to help with cardiovascular health and blood sugar control. It's is a great energy- sustaining food.

❱ PREWORKOUT ❱ POSTWORKOUT ❱ NUTRIENT-PACKED MAINSTAY ❱ GLUTEN FREE
❱ DAIRY FREE ❱ VEGAN

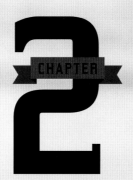

CHAPTER 2

Lunch and Dinner

Lunch and dinner foods are basically interchangeable. The recipes in this chapter are for more substantial meals; they have ingredients that will fill you up for the second half of your day. The balance of protein, healthy fat, fiber, and colorful vegetables will help keep you away from mindless snacking. It's time to upgrade your main meals.

These larger meals are best eaten a few hours before or a few hours after exercise when your body has ample time to digest the nutrients.

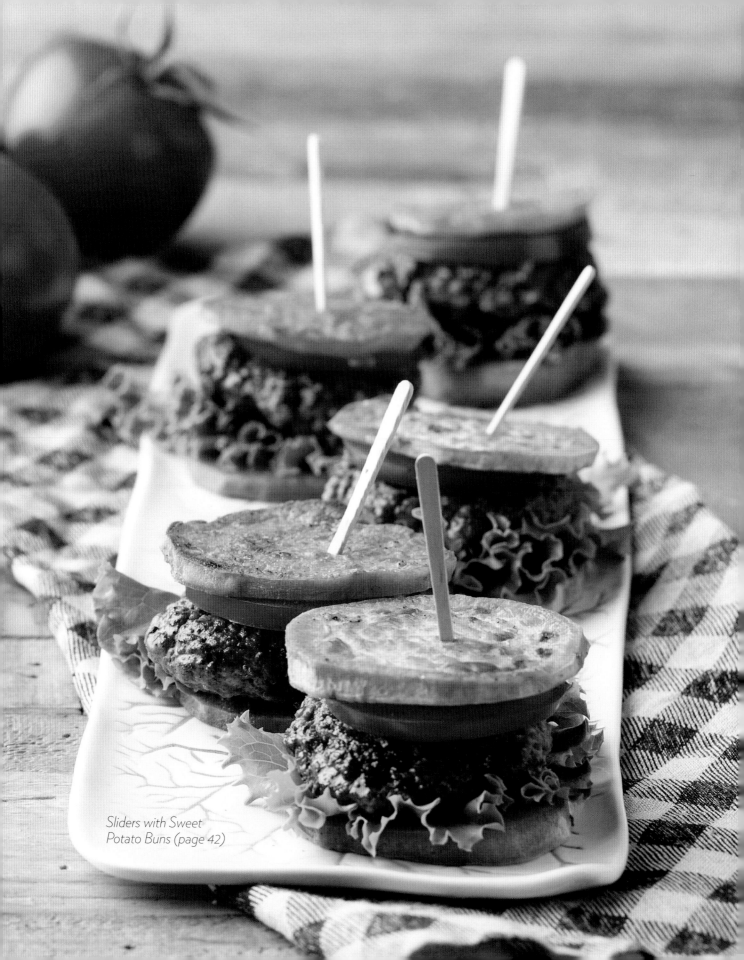

*Sliders with Sweet
Potato Buns (page 42)*

Sliders with Sweet Potato Buns

Sweet potatoes and burgers became a ritual for us after long training sessions. There is something about the combination that brings athletes back to life after a tough workout. This recipe comes from Charlotte Mason of Kaleyeahcatering. com. We are so excited she let us share her most popular recipe! Follow her mouthwatering Instagram @Kaleyeahkitchen.

Buns:

- 2 organic sweet potatoes, at least 3 inches (7.6 cm) in diameter
- 1 teaspoon paprika
  Sea salt and black pepper to taste
- 2 tablespoons (28 g) organic coconut oil or grass-fed ghee

Burgers:

- 1 pound (454 g) grass-fed beef
- 1 teaspoon sea salt
- 1 teaspoon black pepper
- 4 tablespoons (60 ml) olive oil

Toppings:

  Lettuce, tomato, or whatever you want!

Preheat the oven to 400°F (200°C).

Slice the sweet potatoes into ¼-inch (6 mm) rounds and arrange in single layer on a rimmed dark metal baking sheet. Sprinkle with paprika, salt, and pepper. Coat with coconut oil or ghee and bake for 25 minutes or until the edges begin to crisp.

For the burgers, make 4 patties, season with salt and pepper, and drizzle with olive oil.

On a gas grill or grill pan, cook burgers over medium-high heat for 3 to 4 minutes on each side or until cooked through.

Place the cooked burger, lettuce, tomato, onion, and any other toppings between two sweet potato "bun" halves and secure with a toothpick.

Servings: 4 sliders

Notes: These are a great option to bring to a party or potluck. They are bound to be a hit!

Upgrade!
This recipe is a great replacement for **conventional cheeseburgers** or **sub sandwiches.**

DID YOU KNOW? Grass-fed beef, although more expensive than conventional beef, packs in a lot more nutrition. It contains two to four times the amount of omega-3 fatty acids and has higher levels of B vitamins and minerals. It also lacks the hormones and antibiotics of conventional beef.

▶ POSTWORKOUT ▶ NUTRIENT-PACKED MAINSTAY ▶ GLUTEN FREE ▶ DAIRY FREE
▶ LOW FODMAP

Tara's Lean and Mean Turkey Meatballs

Meatballs are the perfect comfort food and bring back memories of childhood spaghetti nights. These turkey meatballs are a lean version of those meatballs, a perfect blend of taste and health. Tara learned in a college food-science class that the addition of prune purée (yes, prunes) helps moisten lean turkey or lean beef. Serve these meatballs with your favorite pasta and sauce the night before an athletic event.

4 tablespoons (60 ml) olive oil

3 garlic cloves, crushed

1 leek, rinsed well and chopped fine

1 egg, lightly beaten

3 tablespoons (45 g) plain yogurt

1 tablespoon (11 g) pure maple syrup or honey

1 tablespoon (11 g) Dijon mustard

2 pitted prunes, chopped extra fine or puréed

2 teaspoons (5 g) Hungarian paprika

½ teaspoon dry mustard

1½ pounds (680 g) ground turkey (or a combination of beef and pork or with sausage)

⅓ cup (40 g) bread crumbs

1 tablespoon (4 g) each, chopped fresh parsley and oregano

Sea salt and black pepper to taste

Add 2 tablespoons (30 ml) olive oil to a skillet over medium heat. Add the garlic, leek, salt, and pepper. Cook for a few minutes, adding a little water to the pan until the leeks are soft. Allow to cool for 5 minutes.

In a large bowl, add the leek mixture, egg, yogurt, maple syrup, Dijon mustard, prune mixture, paprika, and dry mustard, and mix well with a fork.

Add the turkey and ½ teaspoon of salt and mix well. Add the bread crumbs, parsley, and oregano, and mix again.

Form small meatballs with moistened hands or with a large spoon.

In a medium saucepan on medium heat, add the remaining olive oil and brown the meatballs in batches, turning gently until they are brown on all sides and cooked through (test one by splitting it with a fork), about 10 to 15 minutes.

Serve over pasta, or simmer the cooked meatballs in your favorite pasta sauce on low heat and for about 10 minutes.

Servings: 4

Notes: To freeze the meatballs, brown them first in the pan but cook them only halfway. Place the meatballs on a cookie sheet with space between them and freeze for about an hour. Then put the meatballs in a freezer bag; they will keep for up to 2 months. When you are ready to use them, allow the meatballs to thaw for 5 minutes, then add the still-frozen meatballs to a pan of simmering sauce for 10 to 15 minutes.

▶ POSTWORKOUT ▶ NUTRIENT-PACKED MAINSTAY
*Gluten free: Substitute gluten-free bread crumbs.

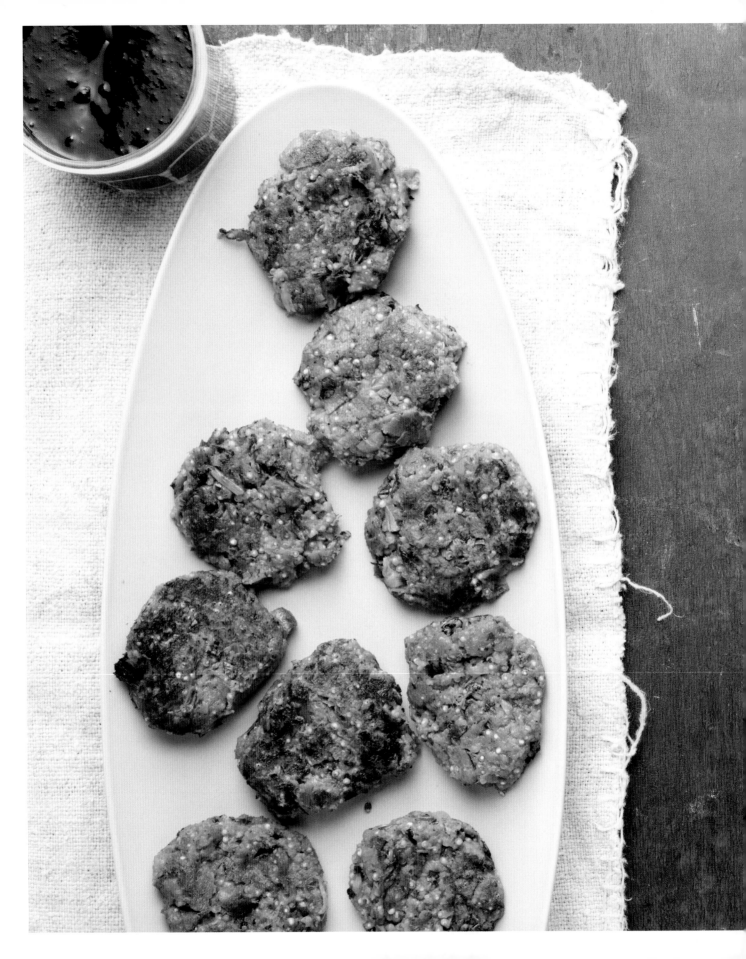

Wally's Sweet Potato Patties with Blueberry Basil Glaze

We made these for our friend Lloyd one night and he couldn't stop eating them. He loved them so much that Tara now makes a batch the last Sunday of every month and shares them with patrons, athletes, and musicians at Wally's, the legendary Boston jazz club that Lloyd and his family run. These patties are a perfect carb-protein combination for sustained energy, muscle repair, and tasty satisfaction.

Patties:

- ½ cup (86 g) cooked quinoa
- 1 tablespoon (15 ml) olive oil
- 1 medium-to-large sweet potato, chopped into large chunks, washed well, with skin on
- 2 large garlic cloves, minced or crushed
- 1 shallot, minced
- 1 leek, rinsed well and chopped fine
- ½ teaspoon sea salt
- ½ teaspoon black pepper
- ½ cup (60 g) bread crumbs
- ½ cup (50 g) shaved Parmesan/Asiago cheese (or either one)
- 2 tablespoons (2 g) fresh cilantro, chopped
- ½ cup (20 g) fresh basil, chopped
- 1 large egg, lightly beaten

Blueberry Glaze:

- 1 pint (300 g) fresh or frozen blueberries (or any berry)
- 1 cup (235 ml) water or maple water
- 1 tablespoon (3.6 g) chili flakes
- ½ cup (20 g) fresh basil, chopped
- 2 tablespoons (40 g) pure maple syrup or honey
- Juice of 1 small lime,
- Sea salt and black pepper to taste

Cook the quinoa in 1 cup (235 ml) of salted water or broth for about 8 minutes. Set aside and fluff with fork occasionally. While the quinoa is cooking, heat a skillet on medium-low heat and add ½ tablespoon (8 ml) olive oil. Add the sweet potato chunks, garlic, shallot, leek, salt, and pepper. Cover and cook for about 10 to 12 minutes, until the sweet potato is soft.

Transfer the sweet potato mixture to a large bowl and mash with a fork. Add the quinoa, breadcrumbs, cheese, cilantro, basil, salt, and pepper and mix together. Add the egg and mix again. Form 4 equal-size patties. Add ½ tablespoon (8 ml) of olive oil to the skillet used earlier and bring to medium heat. Add the patties and cook for 4 to 5 minutes on each side or until the bottoms start to brown.

For the glaze, place all the ingredients in a blender and blend until smooth. Serve in small dish and garnish with extra basil or cilantro.

Servings: 4 patties

▶ POSTWORKOUT ▶ NUTRIENT-PACKED MAINSTAY
*Gluten free: Substitute gluten-free bread crumbs.

Maple~Mustard Glazed Tempeh

Tempeh is a nutritious, fermented, whole-food soy protein that's inexpensive and easy to cook. But it can be a bit bland. Marinate it for a few hours in this simple maple-mustard marinade and bake it until the glaze caramelizes. Jazz up that tempeh!

1 package (227 g) tempeh

2 tablespoons (40 g) pure maple syrup

2 tablespoons (22 g) spicy or Dijon mustard

1 tablespoon (15 ml) olive oil

1 teaspoon chili flakes

½ teaspoon Hungarian paprika

2 tablespoons (30 g) green onions, chopped

1 teaspoon sea salt

1 teaspoon black pepper

Slice the tempeh into finger-size pieces or smaller chunks, if you prefer.

In a bowl, mix together the maple syrup, mustard, olive oil, chili, paprika, garlic, shallot, salt, and pepper.

Place the tempeh slices in a freezer bag and add the marinade, making sure it covers the slices. Allow the tempeh to marinate in the refrigerator for a few hours or overnight.

To cook the tempeh, preheat the oven to 350°F (180°C). Arrange the tempeh in a baking dish or pan and bake for 25 to 30 minutes.

Serve with vegetables and grains or place on top of a salad.

Servings: 2

▶ NUTRIENT-PACKED MAINSTAY ▶ GLUTEN FREE ▶ DAIRY FREE ▶ VEGAN ▶ LOW FODMAP

Lemon~Basil Chicken with Brown Rice Pasta

Pasta dinners and races go hand in hand. Try this delicious and easy-to-make brown rice pasta dish for your next prerace dinner.

1 pound (454 g) boneless chicken breast

4 tablespoons (60 g) olive oil Sea salt and black pepper to taste

5 cups (1.2 L) water

4 cups (400 g) brown rice penne

1 cup (150 g) peas, fresh or frozen

16 leaves chopped basil

4 tablespoons (24 g) fresh lemon juice

Preheat the oven to 350°F (180°C).

Place the chicken on a baking tray and drizzle it with 1 tablespoon (15 ml) olive oil and season with salt and pepper. Roast the chicken for 40 minutes.

While the chicken cooks, bring 4 cups (1 L) of water to a boil in a medium-size pot, add the penne and cook for 11 minutes.

In a saucepan, bring 1 cup (235 ml) of water to boil and cook the peas for 5 minutes. Drain the pasta and peas and place in a serving bowl.

When the chicken has cooled, use two forks to shred it. Add to the pasta and peas with remaining olive oil, basil, lemon juice, salt, and pepper.

Servings: 4

▶ POSTWORKOUT ▶ NUTRIENT-PACKED MAINSTAY ▶ GLUTEN FREE ▶ DAIRY FREE ▶ LOW FODMAP

Mom's Chunky Chicken Chili

This heartwarming chili is filling yet surprisingly light and healthy. The key to a quick preparation is to bake the chicken while you prepare the other ingredients. Rich in protein, fiber, and iron, this chili is a balanced meal that will feed your muscles after a hard workout. It's also a comfort food that's great for a lazy day on the couch watching football with friends. And you probably have most of the ingredients on hand, making it a perfect go-to recipe.

3 cups diced cooked chicken (about ¾ pound [340 g] or 3 to 4 boneless chicken breasts)

1 tablespoon (15 ml) olive oil

1 large yellow onion, chopped

1 medium green pepper, chopped

4 garlic cloves, minced

1 jalapeño pepper, seeded and minced

2 tablespoons (15 g) chili powder

1 teaspoon cumin

1 teaspoon fresh oregano (or ½ teaspoon dried oregano)

½ teaspoon cayenne pepper

2 cups (474 ml) canned, crushed tomatoes

1 cup (237 ml) chili sauce

1½ cups (355 ml) chicken broth

2 teaspoons (10 ml) Worcestershire sauce

¼ teaspoon sea salt

½ teaspoon black pepper

1 can (16 ounces, or 474 ml) black beans, rinsed and drained

1 cup (215 g) white beans, rinsed and drained

Optional toppings:

1 cup (230 g) plain Greek yogurt (will add dairy)

½ cup (80 g) chopped red onion

Preheat the oven to 350°F (180°C).

Season the chicken with a few drops of olive oil and a pinch of salt. Cover with foil and bake for 45 minutes. Remove the chicken from the baking dish and place on a plate to cool slightly. Dice the chicken while it is still warm.

While the chicken is cooking, heat the oil and add the onion, green pepper, garlic, and jalapeño pepper. Cook for 5 minutes on medium heat.

Add the chili powder, cumin, oregano, and cayenne. Cook, stirring occasionally, for 1 minute. Add the chicken, tomatoes, chili sauce, chicken broth, Worcestershire sauce, salt, and pepper. Heat until the mixture is bubbling and cook for 1 to 2 minutes.

Reduce the heat, cover, and simmer for 15 minutes. Stir in the beans. Cook covered for another 5 minutes.

Serve with yogurt and red onions and your favorite sourdough bread, if desired.

Servings: 4

Notes: You can leave out the chicken to make this recipe vegan. Add another cup of white beans and a cup of garbanzo beans to boost the protein.

In a rush? Cut up a store-bought, free-range rotisserie chicken and you will save 45 minutes of cooking time.

It's also easy to double and freeze for a future meal.

▸ POSTWORKOUT ▸ NUTRIENT-PACKED MAINSTAY ▸ DAIRY FREE
*Gluten free: Use gluten-free chicken broth, chili sauce, or Worcestershire sauce.

Roasted Vegetable Mochi Pizza

Mochi is a sticky rice cake made from short-grain rice. We use it to make the crust for this pizza, which has a been a mainstay for team dinners or for dinner the night before a marathon. Delicious, easy-to-digest, and loaded with nutrients, mochi pizza will be a crowd pleaser. Mochi can be found in the refrigerated section of natural food stores.

4	green onions, chopped
1	red pepper, seeded and chopped
1	yellow pepper, seeded and chopped
1	small zucchini, chopped
1	yellow squash, chopped
	Sea salt and black pepper to taste
1	tablespoons (30 ml) olive oil or ghee
1	package mochi

Preheat the oven to 350°F (180°C).

Place the chopped vegetables on a baking sheet, season with salt and pepper, and sprinkle with 1 tablespoon (30 ml) olive oil or ghee. Roast for 15 minutes.

Oil a 9 x 13-inch (23 x 33 cm) pan with the remaining oil or ghee. Cut the mochi into thin strips and place them on the pan, overlapping the strips.

Cover the mochi crust with the roasted vegetables and bake for 12 minutes.

Cool slightly before serving.

Servings: 2

Notes: *Using mochi, ready-to-bake Japanese rice cakes, is an easy way to make a crust that has no preservatives or unhealthy ingredients.*

▸ PREWORKOUT ▸ POSTWORKOUT ▸ NUTRIENT-PACKED MAINSTAY ▸ GLUTEN FREE ▸ DAIRY FREE ▸ VEGAN ▸ LOW FODMAP

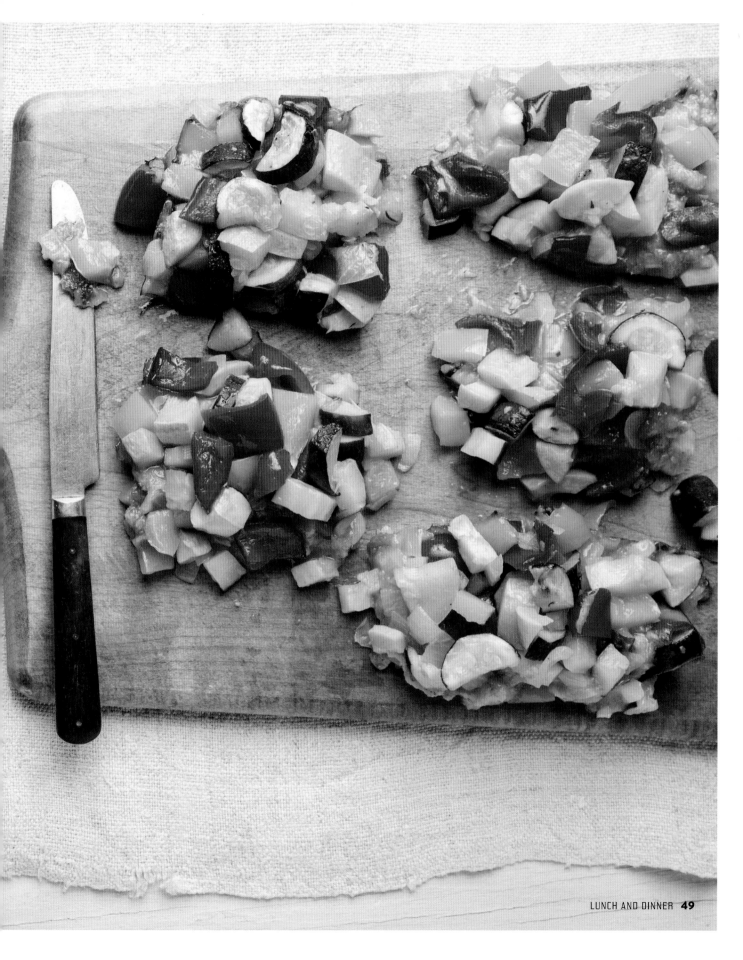

Salmon with Peas and Leeks

Salmon is loaded with protein, anti-inflammatory omega-3 fatty acids, and minerals. This is an easy, delicious meal that will boost your energy, speed your postworkout recovery, and help you focus on your next task.

- 4 pieces (4 ounces, or 115 g) fillets wild salmon
- 3 cups (750 ml) water
- 3 tablespoons (45 ml) olive oil
- 4 leeks, chopped
- 2 cups (300 g) peas, fresh or frozen
- Sea salt and black pepper to taste
- 2 tablespoons (8 g) basil, fresh and chopped
- 1½ cups (190 g) cooked rice (optional)

If you are serving the salmon with rice, rinse the rice with cold water, put it in a saucepan with 3 cups (750 ml) water, and bring it to a boil. Cover, reduce the heat to a low, and simmer for 30 minutes.

Heat 2 tablespoons (30 ml) olive oil in a large skillet on medium heat. Add the leeks, peas, add salt and pepper to taste, and cook for 10 minutes. In another pan, heat remaining olive oil. Season the salmon with salt and pepper and cook it for 4 minutes, skin side down. Turn the salmon over and cook for another 3 minutes.

Add the basil to the leek mixture.

To serve, put the leeks and peas on the plate and place the salmon on top. Serve with a side of rice, if desired.

Servings: 4

Notes: Rice is an ideal add-on after a long workout or on a night before an endurance-based morning workout. On a less active day, decrease the carb content and skip the rice. In a rush? Substitute canned salmon or sardines for the fresh salmon.

DID YOU KNOW? We prefer the rich, orange hue of wild salmon. No matter what fish you choose, it's good to be mindful of seafood sustainability. The Marine Stewardship Council is a nongovernmental organization that provides the world's leading certification for sustainable seafood. For more information, go to msc.org.

▶ POSTWORKOUT ▶ NUTRIENT-PACKED MAINSTAY ▶ GLUTEN FREE ▶ DAIRY FREE

Zesty Zoodles

One night, Tara's training partner and fellow nutritionist, Alicia, brought over a few zucchinis, her spiral slicer (a handy tool that cuts vegetables into spirals, often called a *spiralizer*), and a really good bottle of Spanish wine. The result was creamy pasta noodles, called *zoodles*, without the cream or the pasta— and a few new tracks for their favorite cooking playlist. This low-carb zoodle recipe is a healthy and flavorful take on fettuccine alfredo for those true alfredo loyalists.

Zoodles:
- 3 medium-size zucchinis, cut into spirals using a spiral slicer (or sliced into thin sticks)
- 1 tablespoon (15 ml) olive oil

Cream Sauce:
- ⅓ cup (78 g) extra-virgin olive oil
- ¼ cup (25 g) Pecorino cheese (or Parmesan or Asiago)
- Juice and zest of 1 lemon
- 1 avocado
- 1 garlic clove
- ¼ cup (4 g) basil leaves, stems removed
- 2 cups (300 g) heirloom cherry tomatoes, cut in half
- Sea salt and black pepper to taste

For the sauce, add the olive oil, cheese, lemon juice, lemon zest, avocado, garlic, and basil leaves to a blender or food processor and blend until smooth. Add salt and pepper to taste.

For the zoodles, heat a pan over low heat and add olive oil. Add cut zucchini and cook for a few minutes on low heat until slightly cooked. Remove from heat.

To serve, pour avocado cream sauce over the zoodles. Add sliced cherry tomatoes and mix together.

Servings: 4

Note: *You can find a vegetable spiralizer at a home goods store, a kitchen specialty store, some larger grocery stores, or online. It's not expensive and is a wonderful way to add pizazz to your vegetables.*

"I zoodle so many vegetables that I never buy pasta anymore."
—ALICIA ANSKIS, REGISTERED DIETITIAN, DANA-FARBER CANCER INSTITUTE AT ST. ELIZABETH'S MEDICAL CENTER

▸ POSTWORKOUT ▸ NUTRIENT-PACKED MAINSTAY ▸ GLUTEN FREE

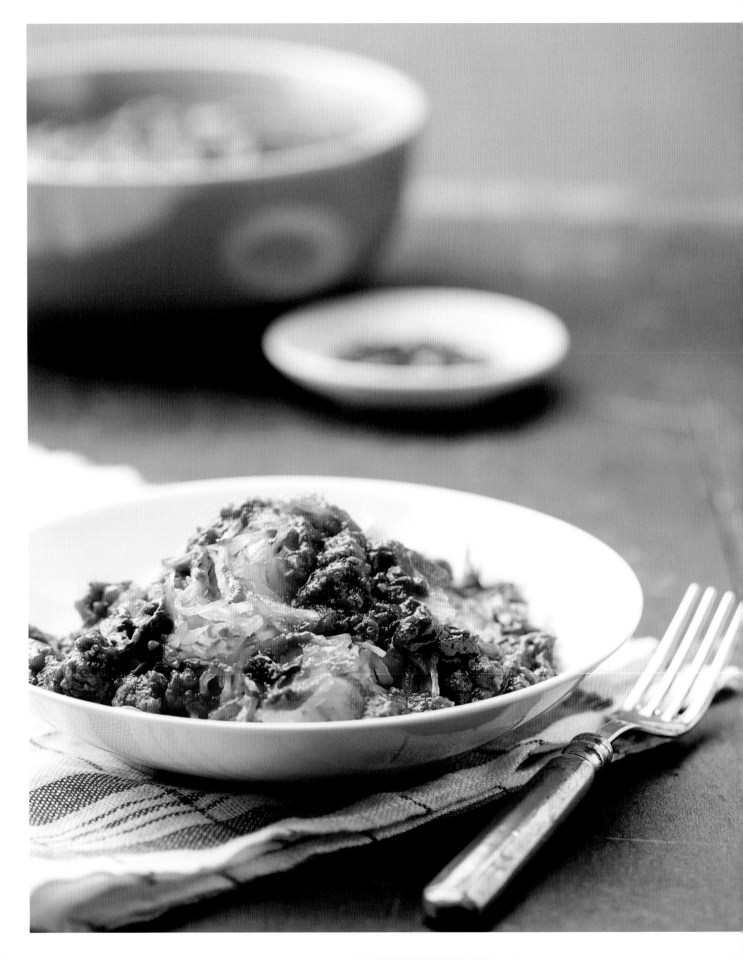

Spaghetti Squash Bolognese

Spaghetti squash is an upgrade from conventional refined pasta because it's loaded with antioxidants such as vitamins A and C. When the squash is cooked, it easily separates into pastalike threads. We use this lighter alternative to traditional spaghetti and meatballs.

2   spaghetti squash

2   tablespoons (30 ml) olive oil

1   onion, chopped

2   cloves garlic, chopped

1   pound (454 g) grass-fed ground beef

2   cans (28 ounces, or 785 g) ground, peeled kitchen-ready tomatoes

4   tablespoons (16 g) fresh oregano (or 2 tablespoons [6 g] dried oregano)

4   tablespoons (16 g) fresh basil

1   cup (225 g) spinach, stems removed and roughly chopped

1   tablespoon (3.6 g) red chili flakes, or to taste

Sea salt and black pepper to taste

Preheat the oven to 375°F (190°C).

Poke holes in the squash with a fork, place them on a baking sheet, and bake for 1 hour.

As the squash cooks, heat the olive oil in a large saucepan on medium heat. Add the onion, garlic, and ground beef to the pan, breaking the up beef as it cooks.

Add the tomatoes, oregano, basil, spinach, red chili flakes, and salt and pepper. Cover and let simmer for 30 minutes.

Remove the squash from the oven. When they are cool enough to touch, cut them in half lengthwise and scoop out and remove the seeds and fibrous layer in the center. With a fork, shred the squash into threads.

Serve the bolognese sauce over your spaghetti squash.

Servings: 4

‣ POSTWORKOUT ‣ NUTRIENT-PACKED MAINSTAY ‣ GLUTEN FREE ‣ DAIRY FREE
*Low FODMAP–friendly: Omit the onion and garlic or use garlic-infused olive oil.

Ten~Minute Madzoon Soup

Madzoon is a yogurt soup, one of Tara's favorite Armenian-inspired recipes. This streamlined version of the soup uses store-bought plain yogurt and is ready in the time it takes to boil the noodles. Tastiest when served lukewarm, this versatile soup can also be enjoyed at room temperature or served chilled on a hot day. Tara eats this as light and refreshing meal a few hours before a race. It's the perfect mix of carbohydrates, sodium, and protein that fuels the muscles, and the mint is a digestive aid that helps calm a nervous belly before the big event.

1¼ cups (125 g) extra-wide egg noodles or gluten-free noodles (measured dry)

2 cups (475 ml) chicken broth

1 cup (230 g) plain full-fat or Greek yogurt

Juice of 2 lemons

⅓ cup (20 g) fresh mint, diced

½ teaspoon sea salt

½ teaspoon black pepper, more as desired

Bring 4 quarts (4 L) of salted water to a boil. Add egg noodles and cook uncovered, stirring occasionally, for about 10 minutes or until done.

While the noodles cook, in a bowl large enough to accommodate the noodles, add the chicken broth, yogurt, lemon juice, mint, salt, and pepper. Stir together until smooth. The yogurt may be clumpy at first, but continue to stir until it's smooth.

Drain the egg noodles, add them to the yogurt mixture, and stir together. The heat of the egg noodles will warm this soup to a lukewarm temperature.

Serve immediately.

Servings: 3 1-cup (328 g) servings

▶ PREWORKOUT ▶ POSTWORKOUT ▶ NUTRIENT-PACKED MAINSTAY
*Gluten free: Use gluten-free chicken broth and gluten-free noodles. **Low FODMAP–friendly: Use a lactose-free plain yogurt.

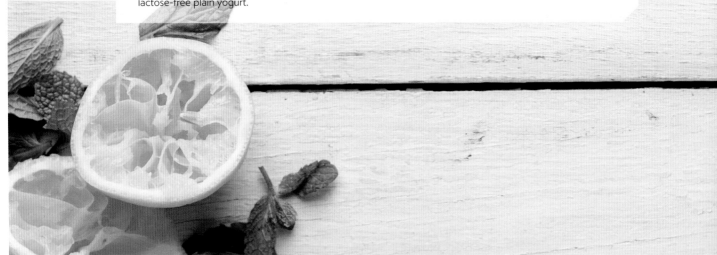

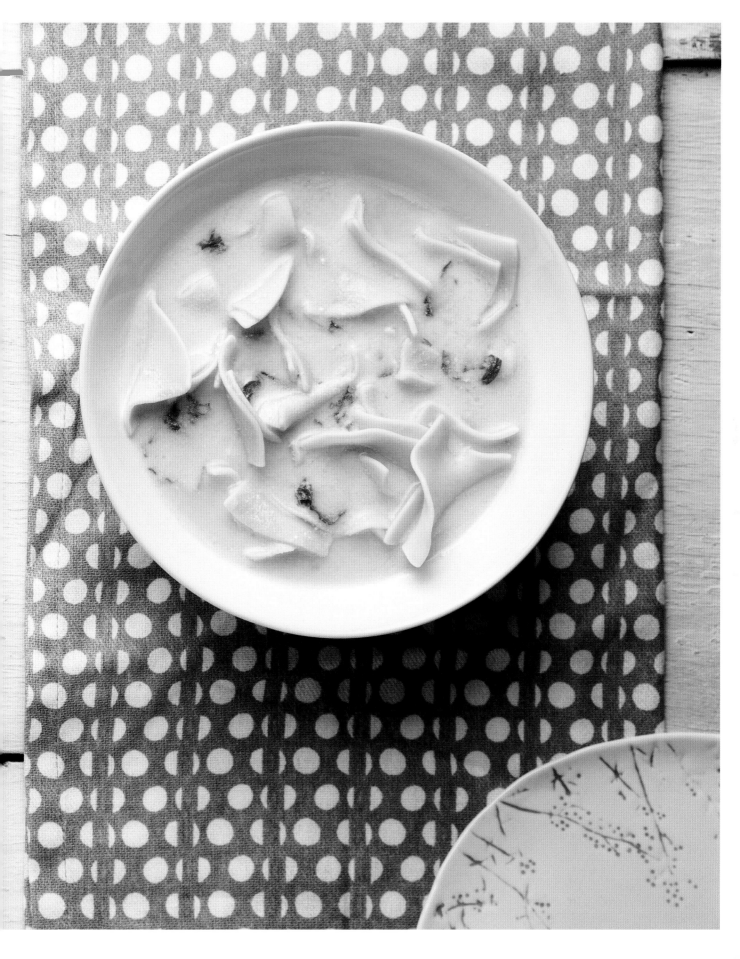

Mat's Easiest Veggie Burgers Ever

When Tara served jury duty, she met fellow juror Mat Schaffer, the James Beard award–nominated former restaurant critic for the *Boston Herald*. Bonded in friendship by a criminal case and further cemented by a deep love for food, Tara and Mat often share favorite restaurant meals and must-have recipes. This is Mat's fail-proof go-to veggie burger recipe.

- 1 can (15.5 ounces, or 450 g) cannellini beans, rinsed and drained
- 2 eggs, beaten (yolks included)
- ½ cup (30 g) parsley, roughly chopped
- ¼ cup (25 g) grated Parmesan cheese
- 2 teaspoons (8 g) Dijon mustard
- ½ teaspoon sea salt
- ½ teaspoon black pepper
- 1 lemon, juiced
- ¾ cup (84 g) toasted bread crumbs (more if needed)
- 2 tablespoons (30 ml) olive oil

Preheat the oven to 375°F (190°C).

Mash the beans with a potato masher or a fork. Fold in the eggs, parsley, cheese, mustard, salt, pepper, and lemon juice. Fold in the bread crumbs, adding more if the mixture is too loose.

Let the mixture sit for 5 to 10 minutes so the crumbs can soak up some moisture, then shape into 4 patties.

Heat the oil in an oven-proof skillet over medium high heat. Cook the patties until they are brown on both sides, about 6 to 10 minutes total.

Transfer the pan to the oven and bake 12 to 15 minutes until the burgers are firm and cooked through.

Serve with your favorite buns or go bunless.

Servings: 4 patties

Notes: *You can substitute black beans, kidney beans, or chickpeas in this recipe, but Mat swears by the cannelloni beans. He serves the burgers on black pepper brioche buns topped with greens, carrots, red onion, tomato, and cucumbers.*

▶ POSTWORKOUT ▶ NUTRIENT-PACKED MAINSTAY
*Gluten free: Use gluten-free bread crumbs.

Fast Split Fish Tacos

Craving Mexican? You can have all the taste of a favorite Mexican meal without loads of cheese, refined carbohydrates, and excess oil. Next time you are craving some Mexican, this speedy recipe is for you.

8 organic corn tortillas

2 teaspoons (20 ml) olive oil or grass-fed ghee

½ teaspoon ground cumin

1 clove garlic, minced

½ teaspoon paprika

Sea salt and black pepper to taste

1½ pounds (680 g) cod, cut into 4 pieces

For topping:

1 avocado, diced

2 bell peppers, diced

½ cup (45 g) cabbage, chopped

1 cup (67 g) fresh cilantro

1 lime, cut into wedges

Salsa, guacamole, or our Guac-Kale-Mole on page 103 (optional)

Preheat the oven to 300°F (150°C).

Wrap the corn tortillas in aluminum foil and place in the oven to warm them.

In a large skillet, heat the olive oil or ghee on medium heat.

Mix together the cumin, garlic, paprika, salt, and pepper. Place the fish in the skillet and sprinkle the spices on top. Cook for 3 minutes then turn and cook for another 3 minutes or until the fish is cooked through.

Put each of the toppings—avocado, bell peppers, cabbage, cilantro, lime, salsa, and guacamole—in a separate bowl for easy serving.

Remove the corn tortillas from the oven and place a piece of fish on top of each one. Add the toppings according to taste.

Servings: 4

Note: *You can use any fish in this recipe, such as ahi or yellowfin tuna or wild shrimp. If you prefer, you can use your favorite meat.*

▶ POSTWORKOUT ▶ NUTRIENT-PACKED MAINSTAY ▶ GLUTEN FREE ▶ DAIRY FREE

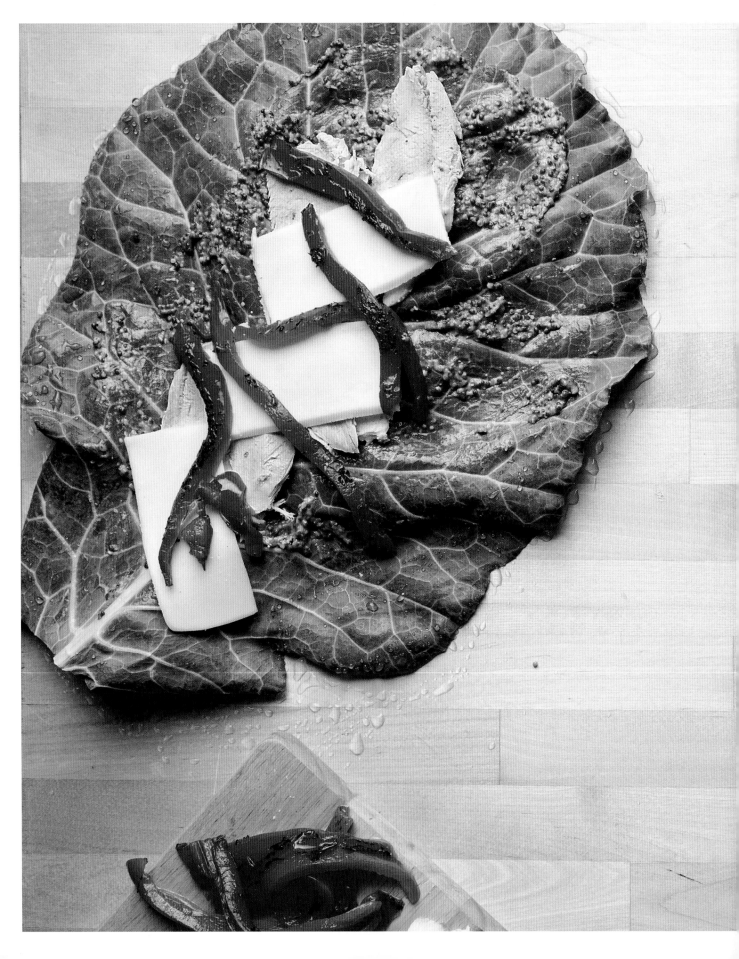

Green Monster Wraps

Picture this scenario: The Jet Blue Park cafeteria in Fort Myers, Florida, spring training home of the Boston Red Sox, on a hot February afternoon. More than fifty young men are hungry for lunch after a long morning of practice.

Tara worked for a decade as the team nutritionist and her goal was to help the players connect with real, and real tasty, food. Sandwiches were always popular and Tara worked closely with the talented FoodZoo catering staff (Chef Shannon, Chef Shorty, and Chef Lee) to help the guys eat for optimal performance. These sandwiches eliminate the traditional nutritionally empty wrap and are covered instead in farm-fresh local collard greens. Without saying anything, the staff put the wraps on the serving line—the vibrant green sandwiches were gone in minutes. Thus, Green Monster wraps were born. What's more, the Sox won the World Series that year. Coincidence?

4 large collard greens, washed well and patted dry

8 ounces (225 g) all-natural cooked turkey, sliced very thin by the butcher

8 teaspoons (36 g) spicy mustard

4 ounces (115 g) mozzarella cheese, cut into 4 pieces (or 4 tablespoons [60 g] hummus)

1 cup (180 g) jarred roasted red peppers, drained of juice

Lay out the collard green leaves on a clean flat surface or cutting board, and spread 2 teaspoons (4 g) mustard (or 1 tablespoon [15 g] hummus) on one side of each leaf.

Place the turkey, cheese, and peppers, evenly divided, on the leaves.

With the leaf lying lengthwise, roll it into a wrap-like sandwich, tucking in the excess along the sides.

Servings: 4

Notes: *Hummus is a great option for this sandwich. Extra-virgin olive oil and vinegar work well, too.*

Blanching the collard greens can help soften them. Simply drop the leaves into a pot of boiling water and remove immediately, shake off the excess water and put them over a tray of ice cubes for a few minutes. Blanching is helpful, but not necessary.

Ugrade!
This is a great replacement for **traditional "spinach" tortilla wraps,** which are green in color but typically contain less than 1 percent spinach. The green color comes from food coloring.

▶ POSTWORKOUT ▶ NUTRIENT-PACKED MAINSTAY ▶ GLUTEN FREE
*Dairy free: Substitute hummus for the cheese. **Low FODMAP-friendly: Skip the hummus.

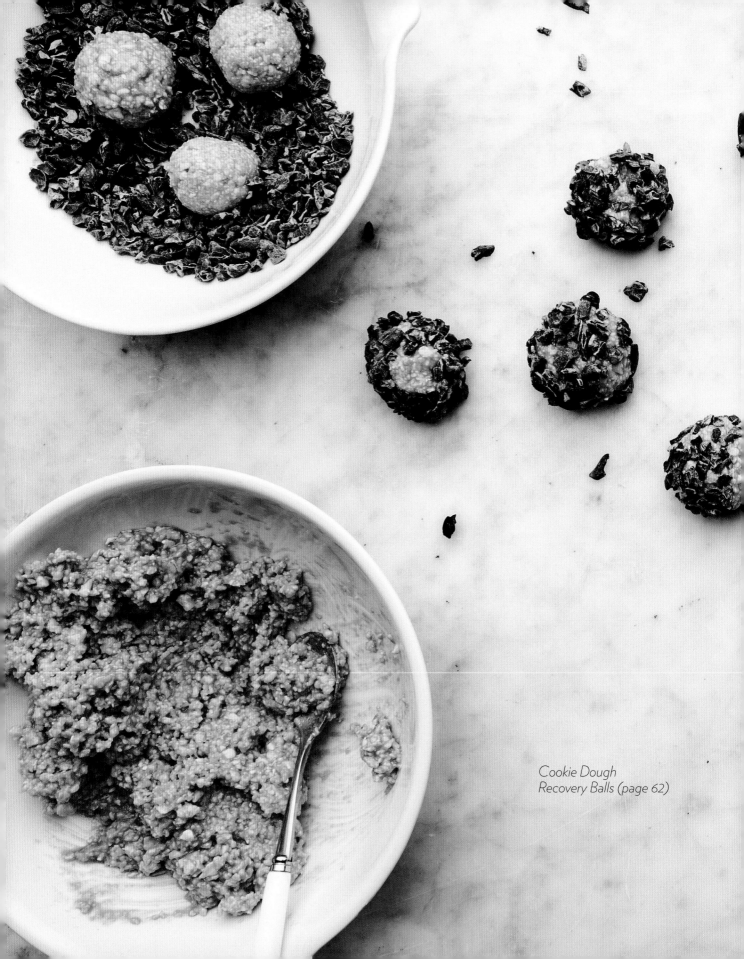

*Cookie Dough
Recovery Balls (page 62)*

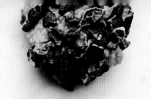
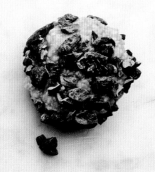
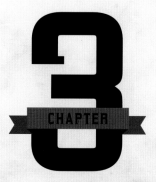

3

CHAPTER

Snacks and Portables

To snack or not to snack? It's better to have a healthy snack on hand than to resort to junky options when you have a craving. If you find yourself hungry, empty handed, and headed for a convenient choice at your office vending machine or corner store, you will most likely find supposedly healthy energy bars that sound appealing—with boasts like "natural" and "high protein"—but with ingredients you have never heard of. The simple solution for the days your body begs for a snack: Choose one of these truly natural and nutrient-packed snacks. The recipes are easy to make ahead of time and the snacks are portable.

Cookie Dough Recovery Balls

Almond Joy Recovery Balls

Micah's BQ Bars

Beet Your Thyme Chips

Cashew Chia Concoction

Panther Mountain Mix

Pistachio Cherry Bites

PR Mochi Bites

Not Your Mama's Cookies

Savory Chickpea Poppers

Sweet Chickpea Poppers

Salty Bananas

Marathon Muffins

Collard Crisps

Cookie Dough Recovery Balls

Remember as a kid reaching into a bowl of raw cookie dough and getting yelled at because of the risk of salmonella? These delicious cookie dough balls taste just as good and have healthy benefits and no risks. Containing protein, magnesium, and the stress-fighting benefits of maca, this treat is easy to make ahead of time and travels well. It is great to eat as a snack after a workout.

1½ cups (340 g) raw cashews

2 teaspoons (5 g) maca

1 tablespoon (5 g) natural brown rice protein powder

4 tablespoons (80 g) pure maple syrup

2 teaspoons (10 ml) vanilla extract

½ cup (87 g) raw cacao nibs or dark chocolate chips

Blend the cashews, maca, protein powder, maple syrup, and vanilla in a high-performance blender or food processor. Do not overprocess; the mixture should have the consistency of cookie dough.

Form 12 balls with the mixture by rolling it between your hands. Roll each ball in cacao nibs or chocolate chips.

Refrigerate or put the balls in zip-lock bags and store in the freezer.

Servings: 12 balls

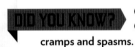 **DID YOU KNOW?** Cashews are an excellent source of the minerals copper and magnesium. Copper helps your joints stay healthy and magnesium helps relieve muscle cramps and spasms.

▸ POSTWORKOUT ▸ NUTRIENT-PACKED TREAT ▸ GLUTEN FREE ▸ DAIRY FREE ▸ VEGAN

Almond Joy Recovery Balls

We were inspired to create recovery balls as homage to our favorite candy bar. These balls are loaded with vitamins, minerals, carbohydrates, and protein to help you recover faster—and lack all the artificial ingredients of their namesake.

1½ cups (215 g) almonds

2 teaspoons (5 g) maca powder

2 tablespoons (10 g) unsweetened shredded coconut

1 tablespoon (5 g) natural brown rice protein powder

4 tablespoons (80 g) pure maple syrup

2 teaspoons (10 ml) almond extract

½ cup (87 g) raw cacao nibs or dark chocolate chips

Blend the almonds, maca, coconut shreds, protein powder, maple syrup, and almond extract in a high performance blender or food processor. Do not overprocess; the mixture should have the consistency of cookie dough.

Form 12 balls with the mixture by rolling between your hands and roll each ball in cacao nibs or chocolate chips

Refrigerate or put the balls in resealable bags and store in the freezer.

Servings: 12 balls

Upgrade!
These two recipes are a great replacement for **cookies, energy bars, or recovery protein bars.**

DID YOU KNOW? All protein powder is not created equal. Look for one that is good quality and does not have additives. Brown rice protein and hemp protein are both good choices. Be wary of whey protein isolate and soy protein isolate powders; they are extracted using chemicals that may be counterproductive to recovery.

▶ POSTWORKOUT ▶ NUTRIENT-PACKED TREAT ▶ GLUTEN FREE ▶ DAIRY FREE ▶ VEGAN ▶ LOW FODMAP

Micah's BQ Bars

Micah is an avid runner and a member of Boston's November Project, a free fitness community, and a *Runner's World* cover model. She's also a nutritionist, a mom, and a vegan. She credits these bars with helping her run fast enough to qualify for the prestigious Boston Marathon on her first attempt. We fell madly in love with her BQ (Boston Qualifier) Bars.

- 1 cup (156 g) gluten-free rolled oats
- ¾ cup (90 g) garbanzo/fava bean flour
- ¼ cup (28 g) coconut flour
- 3 tablespoons (33 g) chia seeds
- 2 tablespoons (14 g) ground flaxseed
- ¼ teaspoon cinnamon

- ¼ teaspoon ginger
- ¼ teaspoon baking soda
- ¼ teaspoon baking powder
- ⅛ teaspoon sea salt
- ⅓ cup (115 g) maple syrup
- ¼ cup (54 g) coconut oil
- 2 tablespoons (32 g) applesauce

- ⅓ cup (115 g) sunflower seed butter
- ¼ cup (42 g) dried cranberries, or dried cherries
- ¼ teaspoon vanilla
- ¼ teaspoon almond extract
- ¼ cup (36 g) almonds, chopped dates (56 g), or walnuts (29 g) (optional)

Preheat the oven to 350°F (180°C).

Grease a 9-inch (23 cm) square pan with a little of the coconut oil.

Combine all the dry ingredients (oats through salt) in a large bowl. Mix the ingredients until thoroughly combined.

Melt the coconut oil in a microwave-safe bowl. In a second mixing bowl, add all the wet ingredients (brown rice syrup through almond extract). Once the wet ingredients are completely mixed, add it to the dry mix. Mix them together and then pour the batter into the baking pan. Add any of the optional items, if you like.

Bake the bars until they are golden brown, about 25 minutes.

Servings: About 16 bars

Upgrade!
These are a great replacement for **energy bars.**

"Not only are these bars easy to throw together and full of unrefined nutrient- dense ingredients, but they are delicious and satisfying. I make them during my marathon training and save a few for the finish line. The week of the big race, I ate almost an entire pan, relying on them for nutrition while traveling and carbo loading. The bars hold moisture and travel well, making them an ideal food for athletes who are always on the go!" —MICAH, DIRECTOR OF NOURISHMENT, LIGHTERCULTURE.COM

▶ POSTWORKOUT ▶ NUTRIENT-PACKED TREAT ▶ GLUTEN FREE ▶ DAIRY FREE ▶ VEGAN

Beet Your Thyme Chips

This recipe will convince you that root vegetables are not dull and flavorless. Edible roots, such as beets, provide many nutrients: fiber, potassium, folate, beta-carotene and other antioxidants. These sweet and savory beet chips will force potato chips to take a back seat.

2 large or 4 medium beets with fresh green tops attached

1 tablespoon (15 ml) olive oil

4 fresh thyme sprigs (dill also works well)

   Sea salt and black pepper to taste

Preheat the oven to 400°F (200°C).

Gently scrub the beets under cool water to remove the dirt, and pat them dry.

Slice the beets into $\frac{1}{16}$-inch slices using a mandolin or slicer.

Arrange the beets on 2 baking sheets and brush them with olive oil. Add thyme sprigs, salt, and pepper.

Bake the beets until the edges brown and curl, about 20 to 25 minutes. The beets will crisp as they cool.

Servings: About 4

Notes: *Beets will stain your fingers and your cutting board. Use disposable gloves and clean the cutting board promptly.*

DID YOU KNOW? **Beets are loaded with nitrates. Through a chemical reaction, the body changes nitrates to nitric oxide, which helps with blood flow and may help you exercise longer and stronger. Cooking reduces the quantity of nitrates, so if you are looking to boost your nitrate intake, try beet juice.**

Wait! Don't toss those beet greens! Beet greens are high in calcium and iron and packed with vitamins A, C, and K. Use them in soups, smoothies, side dishes, or salads.

▶ POSTWORKOUT ▶ GLUTEN FREE ▶ DAIRY FREE
*Low FODMAP–friendly: Substitute two medium sweet potatoes for the beets.

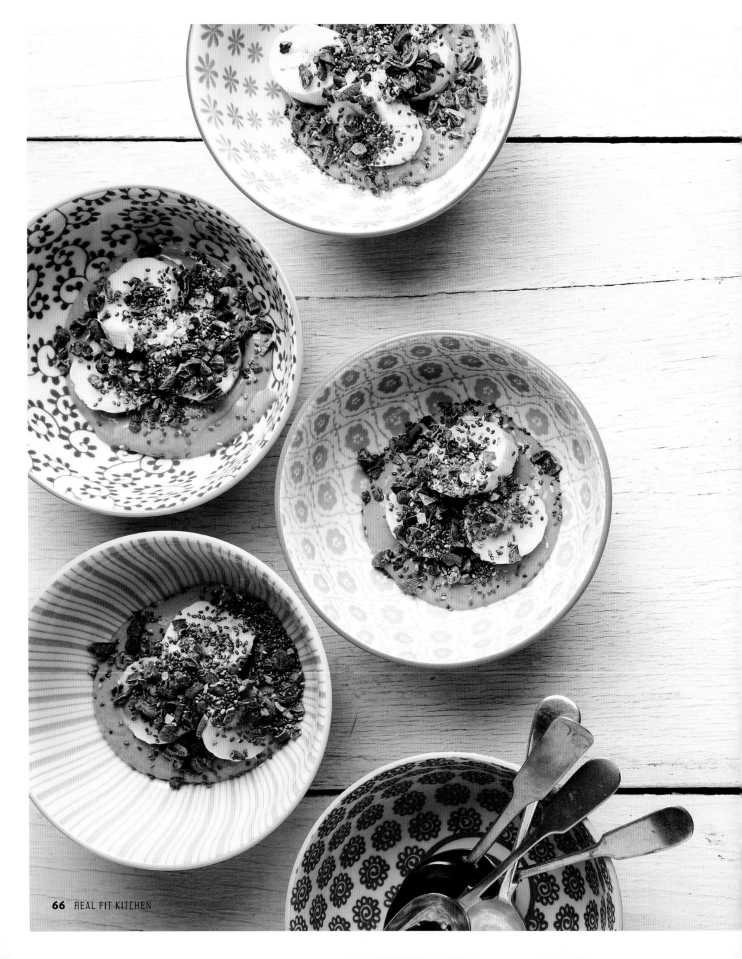

Cashew Chia Concoction

Kate created this recipe when she was traveling for the Texas Half Ironman and it quickly became a staple for her and her training partners. It is fast and easy to make, whether at home or away from your kitchen.

1 banana

2 tablespoons (32 g) pecan, cashew, or almond butter

1 teaspoon chia seeds

1 teaspoon raw cacao nibs

pinch sea salt

Slice the banana into a bowl or cup and add the cashew butter on top. Sprinkle with cacao nibs and chia seeds and sea salt.

Note: Get creative! Top this concoction with two sliced dried figs, ½ teaspoon maca, and ½ cup (115 g) of granola such as our Crunchy Buckwheat Granola (page 39).

Servings: 1

Upgrade!
This recipe is a great replacement for **peanut butter and jelly sandwiches** or **energy bars.**

DID YOU KNOW? Chia seeds have a long history in Mexican and Guatemalan cultures, where people recognized the seeds' ability to increase energy. Known as the "running food," chia seeds are high in omega-3s, protein, vitamins, and minerals. In his book *Born to Run*, Chris McDougall compared the nutritional value of chia seeds to a "smoothie of wild salmon, spinach, and human growth hormone." This wonder seed is an easy way to upgrade your meals!

▶ POSTWORKOUT ▶ GLUTEN FREE ▶ DAIRY FREE ▶ VEGAN

Panther Mountain Mix

Tara's nephews, Trent and Bryce, love to take this flavorful trail mix on their yearly hikes to the top of Panther Mountain, near their family camp in the Adirondacks. Sweet, savory, and chock full of healthy fats, this snack will satisfy for hours. For a hot summer hike, leave out the chocolate chips to avoid a complete chocolate meltdown.

- 1 tablespoon (14 g) coconut oil
- 2 cups (220 g) slivered almonds
- 2 cups (258 g) raw pumpkin seeds
- ¾ cup (110 g) raw sunflower seeds
- 1 teaspoon sea salt
- 1 teaspoon cinnamon
- 6 tablespoons (120 g) pure maple syrup
- 1 cup (120 g) unsweetened dried cherries or cranberries
- 1 cup (175 g) cacao nibs or dark chocolate chips

Preheat the oven to 300°F (150°C).

Lightly coat a large pan with coconut oil.

Spread the nuts and seeds on the pan and sprinkle them with cinnamon and sea salt. (If the nuts or seeds are already salted, do not add salt.) Drizzle with maple syrup and toss to coat.

Bake for 15 minutes and remove from the oven. Add the dried cherries or cranberries, mix well, and bake for another 10 minutes.

Allow the mix to cool, add the cacao nibs or chocolate chips, and mix well.

Servings: About 28 (¼-cup [55 g]) servings

Notes: Pecans, walnuts, and dried coconut flakes will complement the mix, so be creative. It will keep well in an airtight container for about 2 months.

Upgrade!
This recipe is a great replacement for **traditional trail mix or energy bar.**

DID YOU KNOW? Many prepared trail mix varieties are loaded with unhealthy oils, refined sugar, preservatives, and ingredients that won't do your body any favors. Making your own mix ensures that you are getting all the good stuff you want and leaving the rest behind.

"We can't wait to go hiking because we love our Panther Mountain Mix. Can we climb the mountain again?" —TRENT AND BRYCE

▶ POSTWORKOUT ▶ NUTRIENT-PACKED TREAT ▶ GLUTEN FREE ▶ DAIRY FREE ▶ VEGAN
*Low FODMAP–friendly: Substitute 1 cup (100 g) unsweetened banana chips for the dried cherries or cranberries.

Pistachio Cherry Bites

These bites are nutritious and full of fiber, protein, healthy fat, and minerals and are a great source of vitamin E, which helps protect the body against free radical damage caused by stress, environmental toxins, or a super tough workout. These bites are the ultimate proof that what's good for you can taste good, too.

Coconut oil or cooking spray for coating the pan

1 cup (155 g) uncooked gluten-free oats

¾ cup (139 g) uncooked quinoa, rinsed and dried

1 cup (120 g) dried cherries, coarsely chopped

½ cup (62 g) salted, dry-roasted pistachios, chopped

⅓ cup (27 g) unsweetened coconut flakes

2 tablespoons (22 g) chia seeds

1 ounce (30 g) cacao nibs or dark chocolate chips

1 teaspoon cinnamon

½ cup (128 g) unsalted cashew nut butter (almond butter or peanut butter)

5 tablespoons (100 g) pure maple syrup

1 tablespoon (14 g) coconut oil

1 teaspoon sea salt

Preheat oven to 350°F (180°C).

Coat an 8-inch (20 cm) square baking dish with oil or cooking spray and set aside.

Spread the oats and quinoa on a baking sheet. Bake until they are lightly browned, about 8 to 10 minutes. Allow them to cool.

Place the cooled oat and quinoa mixture into large bowl and stir in the cherries, pistachios, coconut, chia seeds, cacao nibs or chocolate chips, and cinnamon.

Combine the nut butter, maple syrup, oil, and salt in a saucepan over medium heat. Bring to a boil and cook for 1 minute, stirring often to prevent burning. Pour this mixture over the oat mixture and toss well to coat.

Pour the mixture into the prepared baking dish and bake for about 15 minutes or until it is lightly browned.

Allow it to cool completely in the baking dish, and then cut it into ½ × 2-inch (1 × 5 cm) bites or 1 × 4-inch (2.5 × 10 cm) bars.

Servings: About 32 bites or 16 bars

Notes: *These portable bites (and bars) will keep in an airtight container for up to 1 week. Bite size, they make a great energy boost or minisnack.*

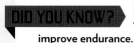 **Pistachios have long been a symbol of health and happiness. They are rich in vitamin E, a powerful antioxidant that, in its natural form, has been shown to improve endurance.**

▶ PREWORKOUT ▶ POSTWORKOUT ▶ NUTRIENT-PACKED TREAT ▶ GLUTEN FREE
▶ DAIRY FREE ▶ VEGAN

PR Mochi Bites

Mochi is an athlete's dream food. Making it into a snack is quick and easy. You can have a puff pastry–like treat with a chewy inside in fewer than 10 minutes. The best part is that mochi is only one ingredient, Japanese sweet rice—no additives or fillers, just rice. Part of Kate's quality carbing before an Ironman race always includes some PR (personal record) Mochi Bites.

1 package mochi, ready-to-bake Japanese rice cakes

4 tablespoons (64 g) nut butter of your choice

1 teaspoon chia seeds

1 teaspoon pure maple syrup

2 teaspoons (10 g) raisins (optional)

Preheat oven to 425°F (220°C).

Cut the mochi into eight 1 × 1½-inch (2.5 × 3.5 cm) pieces. Spread them out on a baking sheet with several inches between them and bake for 8 minutes.

While the mochi bakes, combine the nut butter, chia seeds, and maple syrup and raisins (if you are using them) in a bowl and stir together. Form balls about ¾-inch (2 cm) round with the mixture.

Remove the mochi from the oven. They should be puffed up like a pastry. Slice open the side of the mochi and place a nut butter-ball inside.

Servings: 2

Notes: *You can often find mochi in the refrigerated health-food section of your local grocery store. Check the ingredients to make sure you choose a brand that does not have added sugar or additives like food dyes.*

DID YOU KNOW? **Mochi is a Japanese sweet rice made by steaming the rice and pounding it with large wooden pallets. It is said that Japanese farmers eat mochi to increase their stamina. There are many different ways to eat mochi. Try it! It is a hidden treasures of natural food stores.**

▶ PREWORKOUT ▶ POSTWORKOUT ▶ GLUTEN FREE ▶ DAIRY FREE ▶ VEGAN
*Low FODMAP–friendly: Omit raisins.

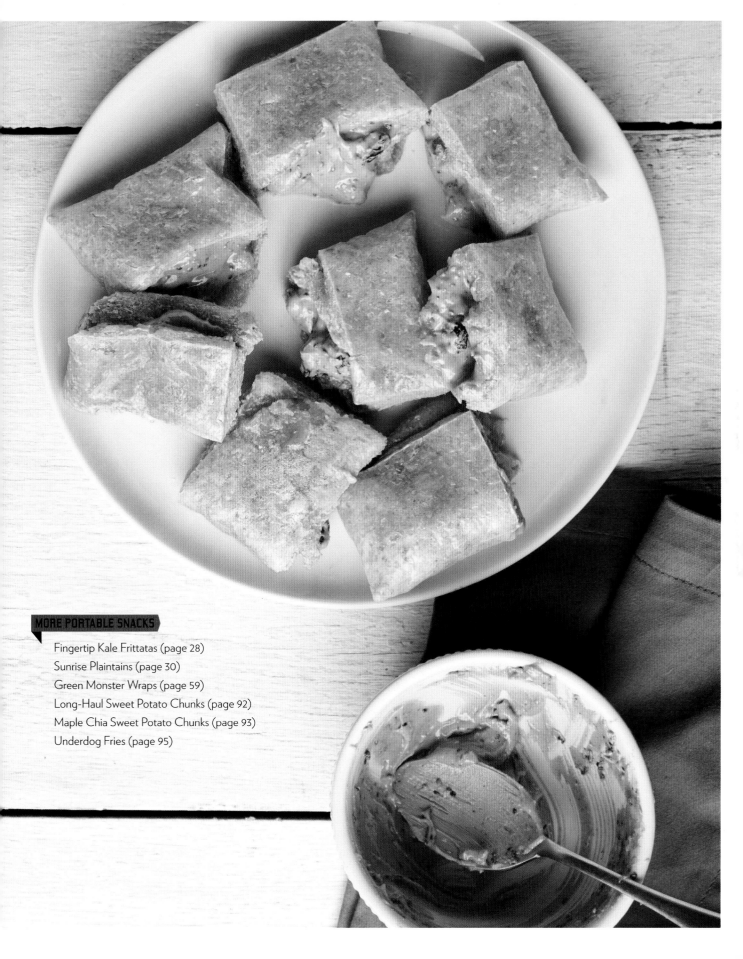

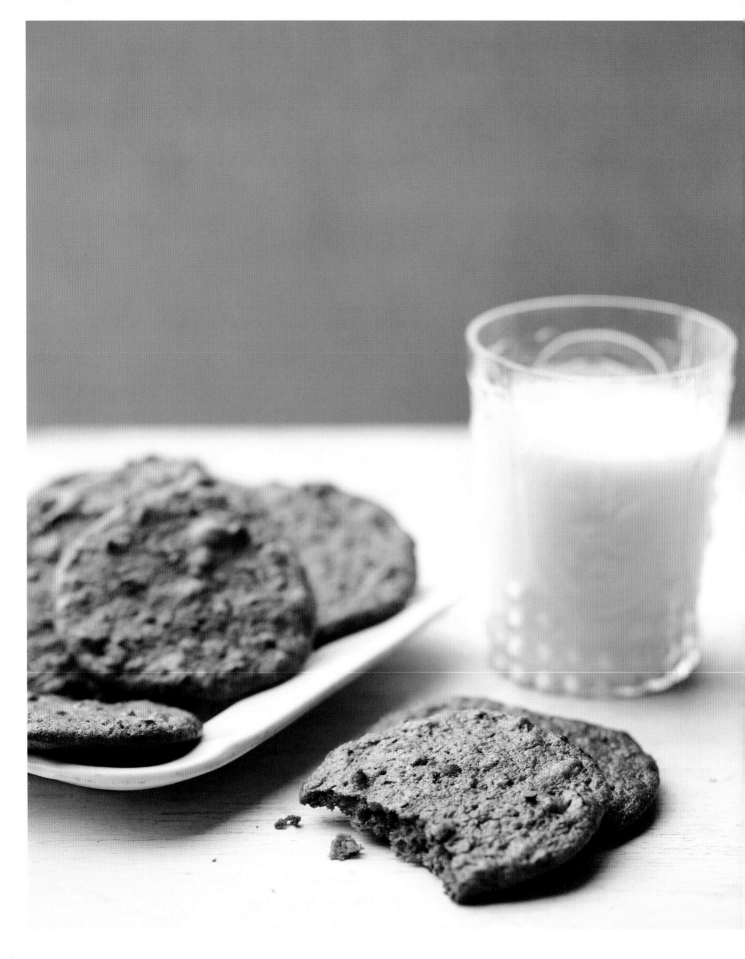

Not Your Mama's Cookies

Athletes love sweet potatoes and cookies. We put the two together to make one heck of a treat. These are perfect for after a workout or to keep you going throughout the day.

Olive oil or cooking spray for the baking dish

2 eggs

½ cup (125 g) sweet potato, baked and puréed, or canned

¼ cup (80 g) pure maple syrup

½ teaspoon vanilla

½ cup (130 g) almond butter

½ teaspoon baking soda

1 teaspoon cinnamon

½ teaspoon nutmeg

½ teaspoon sea salt

1 cup (175 g) cacao nibs or chocolate chips

Preheat the oven to 350°F (180°C).

Coat an 8-inch (20 cm) square baking dish with oil or cooking spray and set aside.

Whisk the eggs. Mix in the sweet potato purée, maple syrup, and vanilla. Add in the almond butter, baking soda, cinnamon, nutmeg, and salt.

Fold in the cacao nibs or chocolate chips.

Form into 12 balls with your hands, then flatten each ball slightly. Space the balls evenly on the cookie sheet. Bake for 30 minutes.

Servings: 12 cookies

Notes: You can substitute canned pumpkin for the sweet potato for a different flavor, but equally nutritious, cookie.

▶ PREWORKOUT ▶ POSTWORKOUT ▶ NUTRIENT-PACKED TREAT ▶ GLUTEN FREE
▶ DAIRY FREE ▶ LOW FODMAP

Savory Chickpea Poppers

Sometimes, you just need a quick and reliable snack food to satisfy a savory craving. These chickpeas will do the trick without leaving you drained like greasy potato chips or crackers tend to do. Imagine a snack that can actually help you control your appetite and stick to smart portions throughout the day and night. These are a win-win.

2 cans (14 ounces, or 392 g) chickpeas, drained and rinsed

2 teaspoons (10 ml) olive oil

2 teaspoons (5 g) ground cumin

2 teaspoons (4 g) ground coriander

1 teaspoon Hungarian paprika

1 teaspoon chili flakes

Sea salt and black pepper to taste

Preheat the oven to 425°F (220°C).

Spread the rinsed chickpeas on paper towels or on a large dish towel and pat dry.

Transfer the chickpeas to a baking pan, drizzle with oil, the spices, salt, and pepper. Toss with your hands to coat evenly.

Roast for 30 to 35 minutes. The chickpeas should be crisp throughout. If they are still soft, roast them for another 5 to 8 minutes.

Servings: 4

Notes: *The poppers are more than a snack. Try adding these chickpeas to salads as well!*

DID YOU KNOW? Rich in fiber and a good source of protein, iron, and manganese, chickpeas help you stay full longer and help stabilize blood sugar.

▶ POSTWORKOUT ▶ GLUTEN FREE ▶ DAIRY FREE ▶ VEGAN

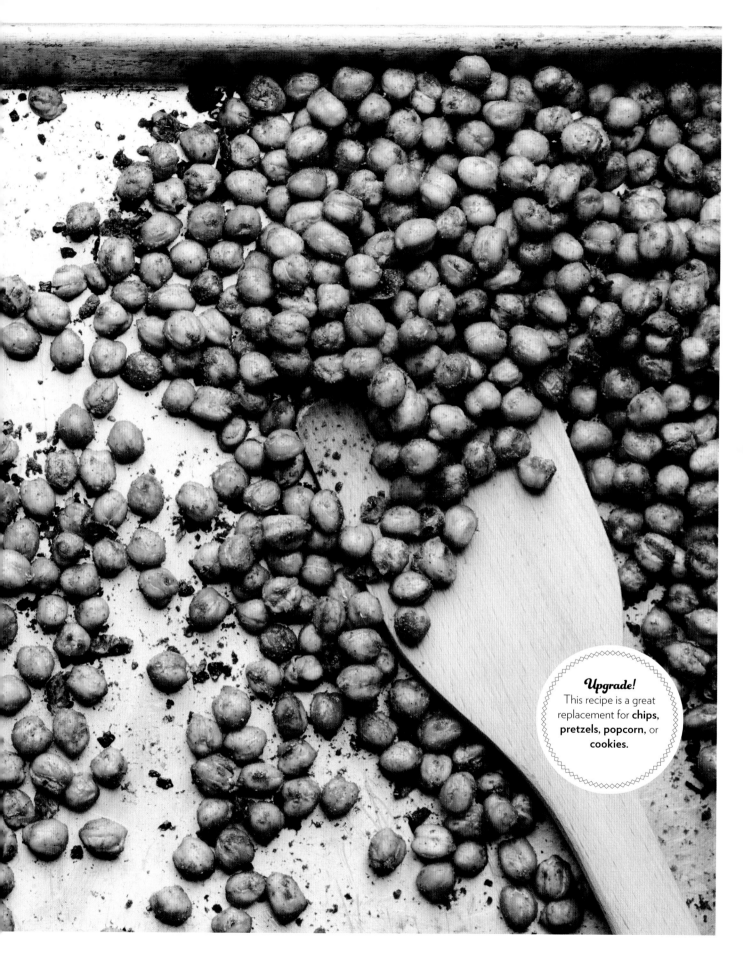

Upgrade!
This recipe is a great replacement for **chips, pretzels, popcorn,** or **cookies.**

Sweet Chickpea Poppers

Here's a sweet version of the chickpea poppers. Sprinkled with a little salt, they are a sweet-meets-savory snack.

- 2 cans (14 ounces, or 392 g) chickpeas, drained and rinsed
- 2 teaspoons (10 ml) olive oil
- 2 teaspoons (5 g) cinnamon
- 1 tablespoon (20 g) pure maple syrup or honey
- Sea salt to taste

Preheat the oven to 425°F (220°C).

Spread the rinsed chickpeas on paper towels or on a large dish towel and pat dry.

Transfer the chickpeas to a baking pan, and drizzle with oil, cinnamon, maple syrup, and salt. Toss with a fork (your hands will get too sticky) to coat evenly.

Roast for 30 to 35 minutes. They should be crisp throughout.

If they are still soft, roast them for another 5 to 8 minutes.

Servings: 4

Notes: *You can change the flavors by using your favorite spices in place of the cinnamon.*

Upgrade!
This recipe is a great replacement for **candy** or **kettle corn.**

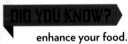

DID YOU KNOW? **When it comes to cinnamon, think outside the baked goods! Cinnamon may help regulate blood sugar and is great to include on a regular basis to** enhance your food.

▶ POSTWORKOUT ▶ GLUTEN FREE ▶ DAIRY FREE ▶ VEGAN

Salty Bananas

Bananas, olive oil, and salt. That's it. Nothing hidden, no chemicals or stabilizers in this simple snack. As a or pre- or postexercise staple, it supplies the electrolytes lost through sweat and is great for athletes who don't like drinking large amounts of sports drinks or other liquids before exercise.

1 banana

2 teaspoons (10 ml) olive oil

1 teaspoon sea salt

Chop the banana into chunks. Mix the olive oil and salt in a small bowl. Add the banana chunks to the salt and olive oil and massage the banana chunks with your hands to coat them. (Then wash your hands really well!)

Servings: 1

Notes: *Take it up notch. Cover the banana with a spoonful of nut butter, spreading it lengthwise. Cover the peanut butter strip completely with crushed tortilla chips. Then slice the banana into bite-size chunks. This is a Bojan Mandaric special, from the uber-fit cofounder of November Project, a free fitness community that's taking over the world. Check it out at november-project.com.*

▶ PREWORKOUT ▶ POSTWORKOUT ▶ GLUTEN FREE ▶ DAIRY FREE ▶ VEGAN ▶ LOW FODMAP

Marathon Muffins

With our hectic schedules, we are big fans of food that we can make ahead of time. It's easy to neglect vegetables when you're always running around so we love these muffins with their extra dose of zucchini. They keep us fueled and help us recover from our workouts.

1 cup (120 g) shredded zucchini

2 eggs

1 cup (100 g) cranberries, fresh or frozen

1 cup (260 g) almond butter

¼ cup (80 g) pure maple syrup

2 teaspoons (5 g) cinnamon

1 teaspoon vanilla extract

½ teaspoon ground nutmeg

¼ teaspoon ground ginger

⅛ teaspoon ground cloves

½ teaspoon sea salt

½ teaspoon baking powder

Olive oil for greasing muffin tins

Preheat the oven to 350°F (180°C).

Shred the zucchini using a cheese grater or by pulsing it in a high-performance blender. Drain the excess moisture by patting the zucchini with several paper towels.

Whisk the eggs in a large bowl. Add the rest of the ingredients to the eggs and stir well.

Grease 8 muffin tins liberally or use muffin pan liners. Pour the batter into the muffin cups.

Bake for 20 minutes.

Servings: 8

Notes: *Try replacing the cranberries with blueberries or apples chunks or another favorite fruit. If you substitute dried cranberries, use ¼ cup (30 g) to keep the muffins Low FODMAP.*

Upgrade!
This recipe is a great replacement for **muffins, bagels, snack foods,** or **breakfast bars.**

DID YOU KNOW? Yes, fresh cranberries are tart! They contain powerful antioxidants and phytonutrients that may decrease the risk of urinary tract infections, improve cardiovascular health, and reduce inflammation. Research has shown that these phytonutrients are more powerful as a complete synergistic group than when isolated. Pairing cranberries with antioxidant-rich zucchini is a powerful treat.

▶ PREWORKOUT ▶ POSTWORKOUT ▶ GLUTEN FREE ▶ DAIRY FREE ▶ LOW FODMAP

Collard Crisps

Collard greens are a tough sell for most people, and we get that. But we promise you won't want to skip this recipe. These collard crisps are a rugged alternative to traditional kale chips and are surprisingly delicious, even making believers out of the skeptics. Packed with nutritious phytonutrients, collard greens are tough enough to stand up to a few flavorful additions without losing their crunch. We could live on these bad boys!

8 collard green leaves, washed well and trimmed of the thick stems

2 tablespoons (28 g) coconut oil, melted

juice and zest of 1 lemon

1 tablespoon (10 g) nutritional yeast

1 teaspoon onion powder

1 teaspoon chili flakes

1 teaspoon sea salt, or to taste

Heat the oven to 200°F (93°C) or set it on the dehydrator setting.

Wash the collard greens well and remove the thick stems. Dry the greens thoroughly, tear the leaves into large pieces, and put into a large bowl.

Mix together the coconut oil, lemon juice, lemon zest, nutritional yeast, onion powder, chili flakes, and salt. Massage the mixture into the collard greens until the pieces are evenly coated.

Line two baking pans with foil or parchment paper and spread out the greens on the pans. Bake for 1 hour, watching carefully to make sure they don't burn. You want them to be dried and crispy. Let cool and serve.

Servings: 4

Note: Store them in an airtight container, and they will keep for 1 week.

Upgrade!
These are a great replacement for **potato chips, pretzels,** and **tortilla chips.**

❱ GLUTEN FREE ❱ DAIRY FREE ❱ VEGAN
*Low FODMAP–friendly: Omit the onion powder.

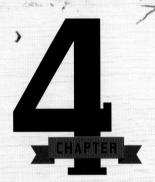

4

CHAPTER

Vegetables and Salads

We know we should be eating more vegetables and salads. But somehow, conventional sports nutrition advice has lost focus on the importance of eating a meal that emphasizes the potential power of vegetables. If we consume the amount of calories that will sustain us, but eat food devoid of the proper nutrients, our body will fatigue much faster. As athletes, we go through these nutrients faster than the average person so, in this chapter, we include flavorful and nutrient-packed recipes that will not only help strengthen your body but will leave you wanting more!

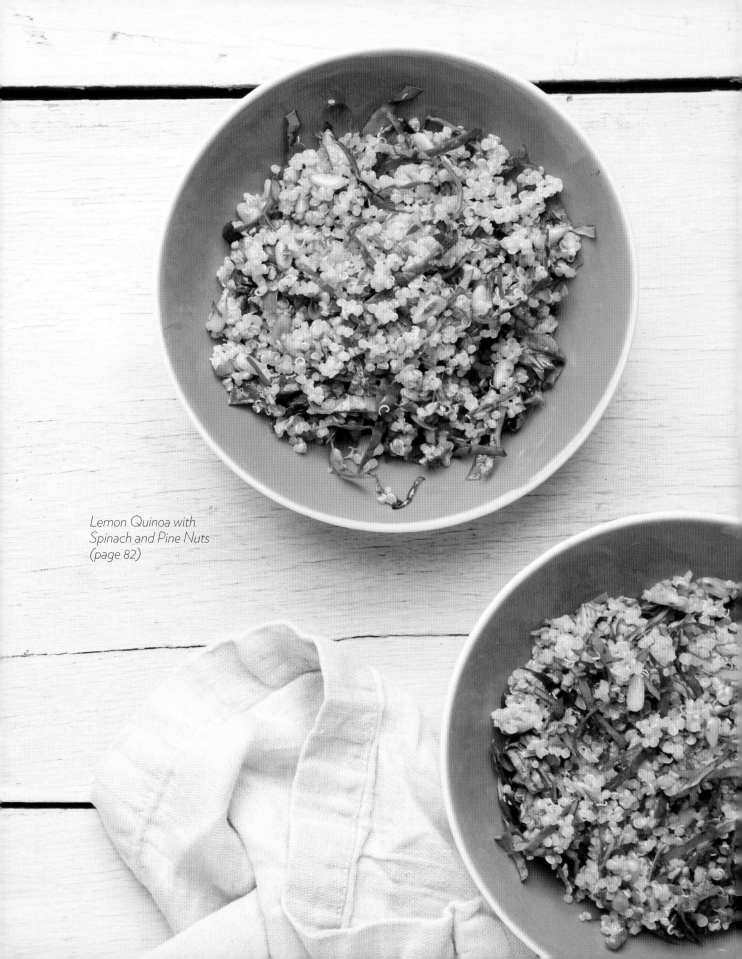

Lemon Quinoa with
Spinach and Pine Nuts
(page 82)

Lemon Quinoa with Spinach and Pine Nuts

Quinoa has a high nutritional profile—it's gluten free and full of protein, B vitamins, iron, zinc, potassium, calcium, and vitamin E—and it cooks more quickly than any other grain. Spinach and parsley add even more nutritional benefits to this dish. This recipe, easy to make and delicious, was created by nutrition expert, marathoner, and yogi, Elise Museles at Kale and Chocolate. Check out her website at kaleandchocolate.com.

- 1 cup (173 g) quinoa
- 2 cups (475 ml) water (or use 1 cup water and 1 cup vegetable broth for more flavor)
- 1 teaspoon sea salt (if you are not using broth)

- 2 cups (225 g) raw spinach
- ¼ cup (30 g) fresh flat leaf parsley
- ¼ cup (70 g) pine nuts, toasted
- 2 teaspoons (4 g) grated lemon zest

- ¼ cup (60 ml) fresh lemon juice
- 1 teaspoon ground cumin
- Sea salt and black pepper to taste
- ¼ cup (60 ml) olive oil

Preheat the oven to 350°F (180°C).

Rinse the quinoa in a bowl of water and drain it. Transfer it to a saucepan, add the salt and 2 cups (470 ml) water (or 1 cup [235 ml] broth and 1 cup [235 ml] water), and bring it to a boil. Cover, reduce the heat and simmer for 15 minutes or until all the water is absorbed. Let the quinoa sit covered for an additional 5 minutes before removing the lid. Allow the quinoa to cool for at least 20 minutes. While the quinoa is cooking and cooling, thinly slice the spinach and chop the parsley.

Place the pine nuts on a baking sheet and toast them in the oven for 8 minutes.

Put the cooled quinoa in a serving bowl, add the toasted pine nuts, lemon zest, and parsley, and mix together. Place the sliced, raw spinach on top of the quinoa.

In a separate bowl, whisk together the lemon juice, cumin, salt, and pepper. Drizzle in olive oil. Pour the dressing to the top of the bowl to moisten all the ingredients. Salt and pepper to taste.

Servings: 6

DID YOU KNOW? If you soak grains before you cook them, your body can absorb more of the nutrients because soaking removes a lot of the phytic acid that blocks mineral absorption. Allow them to sit in a bowl of cold water for up to 8 hours before cooking. You can also find prerinsed grains at some grocery and health food stores.

▶ POSTWORKOUT ▶ NUTRIENT-PACKED MAINSTAY ▶ GLUTEN FREE ▶ DAIRY FREE ▶ VEGAN
▶ LOW FODMAP

Show Me the Greens

We encourage athletes to have greens on hand. Loaded with nutrients like chlorophyll, lutein, and beta-carotene, greens are low in calories and can help replenish nutrients after a workout, improve your immune system, and help you perform your best every day. We are sure you will see performance gains by adding more greens to your plate.

- 8 cups (536 g) greens (kale, collards, mustard greens, spinach, beet greens, bok choy or a mixture)
- 1 clove garlic, minced
- 2 tablespoons (30 ml) olive oil
- 1 teaspoon sea salt, or to taste
- 1 teaspoon red pepper flakes, or to taste

Heat the oil in a large skillet over medium heat. Add the greens and stir.

Wash the greens thoroughly under running water to remove any sand or grit and remove the thick center stems. Tear or cut them into large pieces.

Add the garlic, salt, and pepper flakes, and continue to stir for 3 to 4 minutes.

Servings: 2

DID YOU KNOW? It is a good idea to mix up your greens and try different ones. Each green is unique and has vital nutrients.

Greens contain the antioxidant alpha-lipoic acid which can help defend against oxidative assaults from strenuous training and from everyday aging.

▶ NUTRIENT-PACKED MAINSTAY ▶ GLUTEN FREE ▶ DAIRY FREE ▶ VEGAN
*Low FODMAP–friendly: Omit the garlic or use garlic-infused olive oil.

Bostonian Brussels Sprouts

Just the words "brussels sprouts" brings back the images of those mushy green things from childhood. But these roasted sprouts are crisp and delicious, rich in antioxidants, help with muscle repair, and boost overall health. Folate, vitamin C, vitamin A, and lots of phytonutrients work together to make this one powerful little vegetable.

5 cups (440 g) Brussels sprouts

2 cups (340 g) sliced fresh pears (any variety), skin on

¼ cup (25 g) raw pecans

1 cup (100 g) cranberries, fresh or frozen

Sea salt and black pepper to taste

3 tablespoons (45 ml) olive oil

Preheat the oven to 350°F (180°C).

Cut the bottoms off the brussels sprouts and cut them in half.

Combine the halved brussels sprouts, pear slices, pecans, cranberries, and salt and pepper on a baking sheet and drizzle with the olive oil.

Roast for 35 to 40 minutes.

Servings: 4

▶ NUTRIENT-PACKED MAINSTAY ▶ GLUTEN FREE ▶ DAIRY FREE ▶ VEGAN

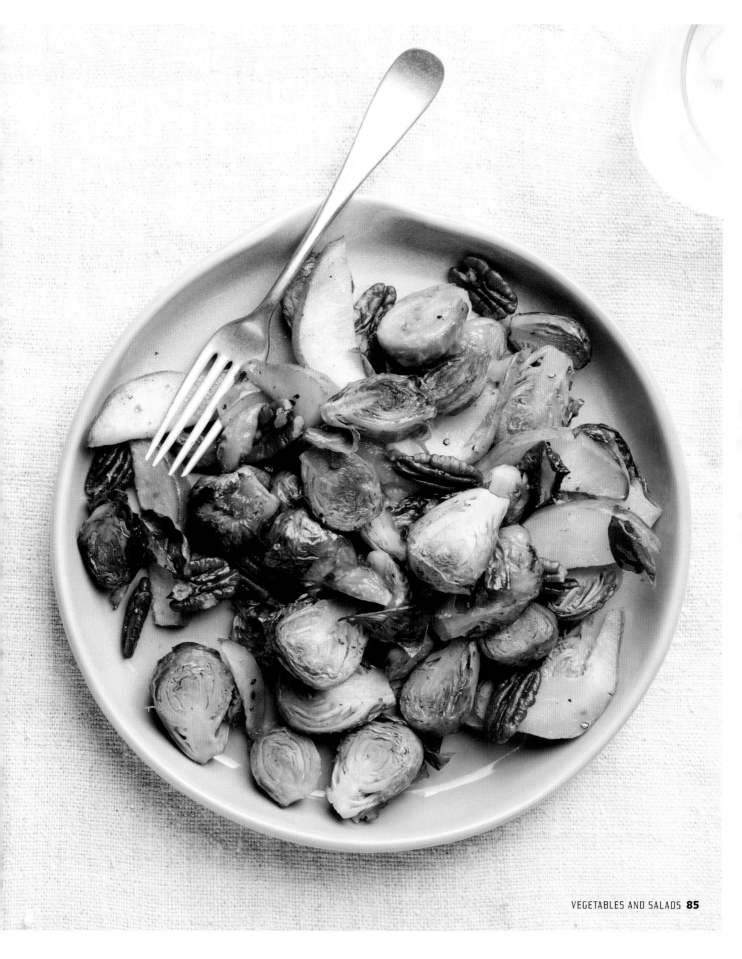

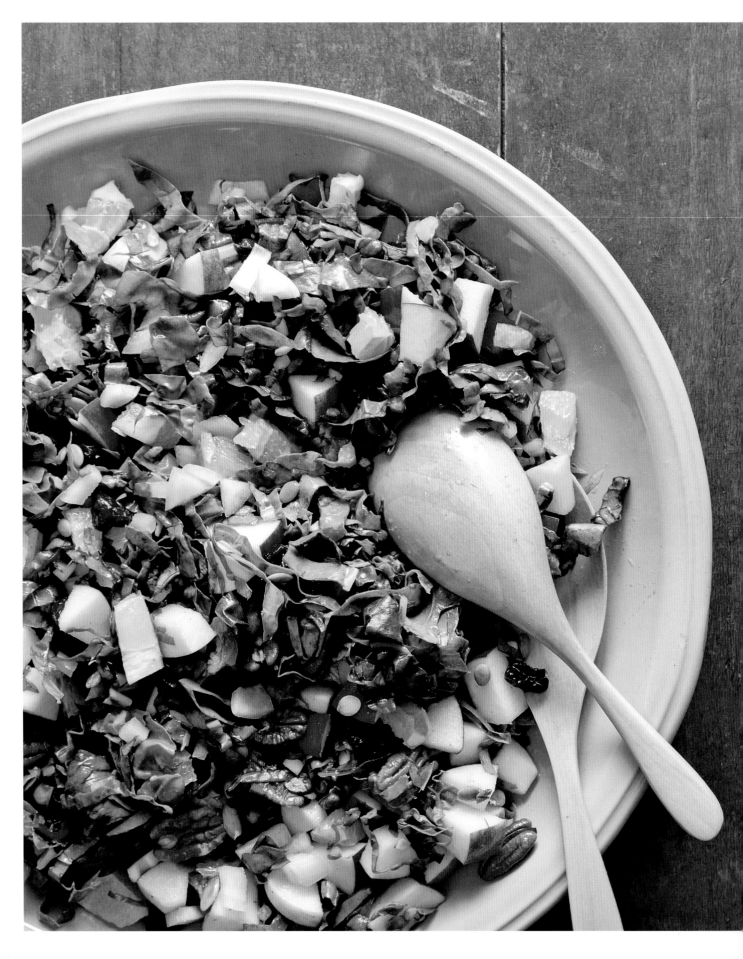

Rainbow Chard Salad

This colorful salad impresses even the pickiest vegetable eaters. Chard is a great source of antioxidant phytonutrients. One phytonutrient group found in chard is called *betalains* which have been shown to provide significant antioxidant, anti-inflammatory, and detoxification support. Though exercise is healthy for you, it is a stressor to the body, so it is important to help support detoxification through foods like swiss chard.

6 cups (400 g) swiss chard: red, green, or rainbow, sliced into thin ribbons

2 oranges, chopped

1 small onion, chopped

1 apple, chopped

½ cup (50 g) raw pecans

⅓ cup (44 g) raw pepitas

3 tablespoons (30 g) dried cherries

⅓ cup (60 g) pomegranate seeds (optional)

For the Dressing:

2 tablespoons (30 ml) unfiltered, apple cider vinegar

1 tablespoon (20 g) pure maple syrup

2 tablespoons (30 ml) olive oil

⅓ teaspoon sea salt

⅓ teaspoon black pepper

⅛ teaspoon turmeric powder

⅛ teaspoon cayenne

Combine all the salad ingredients in a large salad bowl.

Combine all ingredients for the dressing in a small bowl or a bottle and mix together.

Pour the dressing on the salad and toss.

Servings: 4

Notes: *Pomegranate seeds are a great addition to this salad. They are delicious and full of antioxidants. We made them optional because it is time consuming to pick them out of the fruit and it can be expensive to purchase the seeds alone. This recipe can be made into an entrée salad by adding some diced chicken, tempeh, fish, egg, or strips of beef.*

▶ POSTWORKOUT ▶ NUTRITION-PACKED MAINSTAY ▶ GLUTEN FREE ▶ DAIRY FREE ▶ VEGAN

Out~of~Town Carrots

Carrots are delicious as is, but this recipe adds Mediterranean spices for a punch of flavor that complements their natural sweetness. Trying to use up a few carrots before leaving for a holiday trip, Tara created this recipe by experimenting with her favorite spice blends. Cooking the carrots in a slow cooker for a few hours to let the flavors marinate works well but so does cooking the carrots on the stove for 10 minutes. Kate loves these after a long session in the pool.

4	large carrots
1	large onion
1	cup (235 ml) gluten-free chicken broth
1	teaspoon tomato paste
2	tablespoons (30 ml) olive oil (stove top method)
¼	cup (85 g) pure maple syrup
2	tablespoons (12 g) Baharat spice blend
½	teaspoon Hungarian paprika
1	teaspoon Aleppo chili flakes
2	cloves of garlic (optional)
	Sea salt and black pepper to taste
⅓	cup (40 g) dried cherries
2	sprigs of fresh thyme for garnish (optional)

Wash carrots well. No need to peel them.

Slice carrots into ½-inch (1.3 cm) thick disks.

In a slow cooker:

Chop the onion into large slices and put them into the slow cooker along with the carrots and chicken broth, tomato paste, maple syrup, spices, garlic, salt and pepper.

Cook on high for 2 hours, stirring occasionally.

Add the dried cherries in the last half hour of cooking so they don't get soggy.

On the stove top:

Bring a large pot of water to boil. Have a bowl of ice and water nearby.

Whisk together 1 tablespoon (15 ml) olive oil and the honey or maple syrup and set aside in small bowl.

Add the carrots to boiling water and cook until tender but still crisp, about 5 minutes.

Remove the carrots, and put them in the ice bath to stop the cooking. Let them cool for a few minutes, remove them from ice bath and allow them to dry on a towel for 5 minutes.

In a saucepan over low heat, cook the garlic in 1 tablespoon (15 ml) olive oil. Add the chicken broth and tomato paste, stir. Add the spices and dried cherries, and stir together.

Add the carrots and mix all of the ingredients together, sauté for about 8 minutes. Garnish with thyme, if desired.

Servings: 2 to 4

▶ GLUTEN FREE ▶ DAIRY FREE ▶ VEGAN

Arugula with Cherries and Pepitas

This salad is so simple, it requires hardly any preparation time. Use baby spinach or kale in place of the arugula, depending on what's freshest. Pepitas (a.k.a. pumpkin seeds) are a good source of iron and zinc, a combination that helps the formation of red blood cells, which carry oxygen to the muscles.

6 cups (120 g) baby arugula, torn into bite-size pieces

⅔ cup (87 g) raw pepitas

⅔ cup (67 g) dried cherries or cranberries

For the dressing:

4 tablespoons (60 ml) olive oil

2 tablespoons (30 ml) lemon juice, freshly squeezed

Sea salt and black pepper to taste

2 teaspoons (10 g) pure maple syrup (optional)

Combine all the salad ingredients in a large salad bowl.

Combine all ingredients for the dressing in a small bowl or jar and mix together.

Pour the dressing on the salad and toss.

Servings: 4

Note: *You can also make this with fresh berries.*

▶ NUTRITION-PACKED MAINSTAY ▶ GLUTEN FREE ▶ DAIRY FREE

Lazy Beans

These green beans take 5 minutes to prepare. We don't even use a fork to eat them. Of course, they can also complement a beautiful dinner. Green beans contain a wide variety of health-promoting antioxidants, including carotenoids and flavonoids. From eye health to heart health, green is good.

¼ cup (60 ml) water

1 pound (500 g) fresh haricot vert (tiny green beans), rinsed well and with the rough ends trimmed

Juice of 1 lemon (or 2 to 3 tablespoons lemon juice)

½ teaspoon of sea salt

Place water in a medium pan and heat on medium heat. Add the green beans. Cook for about 1 minute. Add the lemon juice and cook for 1 minute.

Remove from the heat. The beans should be bright green and crunchy. We like them ever so slightly cooked or steamed. Sprinkle salt on top.

Servings: 4

Notes: *As a shortcut, you can use prewashed, pretrimmed green beans (give them a good rinse anyway) and bottled lemon juice.*

▶ GLUTEN FREE ▶ DAIRY FREE ▶ VEGAN ▶ LOW FODMAP

OmGal's Soulful Salad

Rebecca Pacheco, a Boston-based yoga teacher, author, and avid runner shares our love of good food to fuel an active body. Her salad contains kale, the most fashionable vegetable on the planet, our cruciferous crush, and the darling of any farmers' market. For Rebecca, of Portuguese descent, kale was a humble staple in her childhood meals, prepared by her Vavo (grandmother). This shredded kale salad is a yoga teacher's go-to comfort food. For more on yoga, running, and mindfulness, check out omgal.com and her book, *Do Your Om Thing*.

1   tablespoon (15 ml) olive oil
    Juice of ½ fresh lime
½   teaspoon sea salt
½   teaspoon black pepper
    Cayenne pepper,
    to taste
1   large bunch kale, washed,
    stems removed

Mix together the olive oil, lime juice, salt, pepper, and cayenne pepper if desired, in a small bowl. Set aside.

Layer the kale leaves like sheets of paper into small stacks. Roll a stack of leaves as if you were rolling up a sleeping bag. Slice the kale, as thinly as possible, to create very fine ribbons of kale that you'll be able to twirl around your fork like noodles. Continue cutting each stack.

With your hands, massage the oil mixture into the kale. This helps soften the kale so it better absorbs the citrus and spice.

Servings: 2

Notes: *Raw kale can be tough and dry, but slicing it into very fine strips, called* chiffonade, *makes it more pleasant to eat.*

Add a fiber-rich grain such as bulgur or quinoa and your favorite lean protein and you have a complete meal.

▶ NUTRIENT-PACKED MAINSTAY ▶ GLUTEN FREE ▶ DAIRY FREE ▶ VEGAN ▶ LOW FODMAP

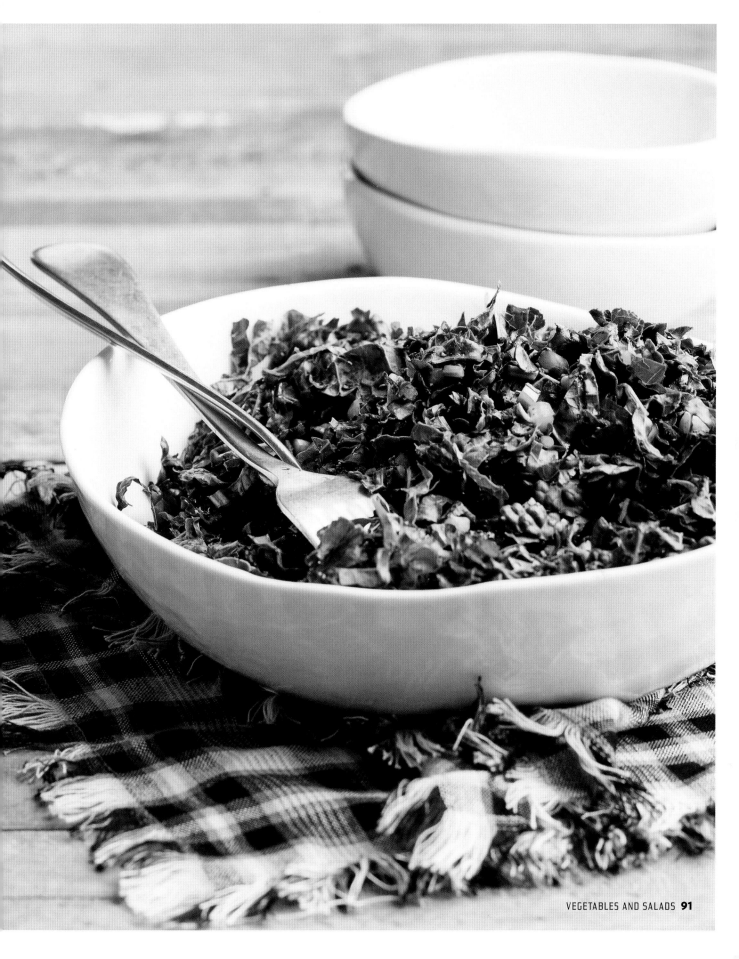

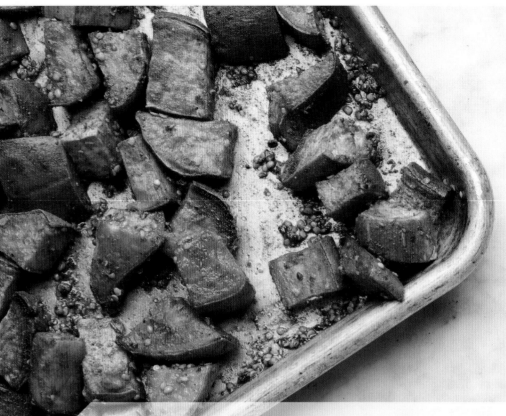

Long~Haul Sweet Potato Chunks

You may turn orange with our spicy take on sweet potato fries. These chunks provide long-lasting energy for a few hours before an upcoming endurance event or as part of your muscle fuel after exercise recovery plan. Dusted with additional anti-inflammatory spices and healthy fats, these little chunks are powerful.

2 large sweet potatoes, washed well, skin on

1½ tablespoons (21 g) coconut oil

1 tablespoon (6.8 g) ground turmeric

1 tablespoon (5 g) hemp seeds

1 teaspoon cumin

1 tablespoon (18 g) sea salt

1 teaspoon black pepper

Preheat the oven to 350°F (180°C). Line a baking sheet with aluminum foil or grease it with a small amount of olive oil.

Cut the sweet potatoes into small chunks and place in medium-size bowl.

Add coconut oil, turmeric, hemp seeds, cumin, salt, and black pepper. Massage the oil and spices onto the sweet potatoes with your hands.

Bake for 40 minutes or until the outsides are light brown and the insides are tender. Turn the chunks at 20 minutes.

Servings: 2

Upgrade!
This recipe is a great replacement for **french fries, tater tots, mashed potatoes,** or **hash browns.**

▶ PREWORKOUT ▶ POSTWORKOUT ▶ GLUTEN FREE ▶ DAIRY FREE ▶ VEGAN ▶ LOW FODMAP

Maple Chia Sweet Potato Chunks

Try these sweet potato chunks with a sweet spin.

Olive oil (optional)

2 large sweet potatoes, washed well, no need to remove the skin

1½ tablespoons (21 g) coconut oil

1 tablespoon (18 g) sea salt

1 tablespoon (20 g) pure maple syrup

1 tablespoon (11 g) chia seeds

2 teaspoons (4.6 g) cinnamon

Preheat the oven to 350°F (180°C). Line a baking sheet with aluminum foil or grease it with a small amount of olive oil.

Cut the sweet potatoes into nugget-size chunks. Place in medium-size bowl. Add the coconut oil, salt, maple syrup, chia seeds, and cinnamon. Massage the oil and spices into the sweet potatoes with your hands.

Bake for 40 minutes or until the outsides are light brown and the insides are tender. Turn the chunks at 20 minutes.

Servings: 2

Upgrade!
This recipe is a great replacement for **french fries** or **kettle corn.**

❱ PREWORKOUT ❱ POSTWORKOUT ❱ NUTRIENT-PACKED TREAT ❱ GLUTEN FREE ❱ DAIRY FREE
❱ VEGAN ❱ LOW FODMAP

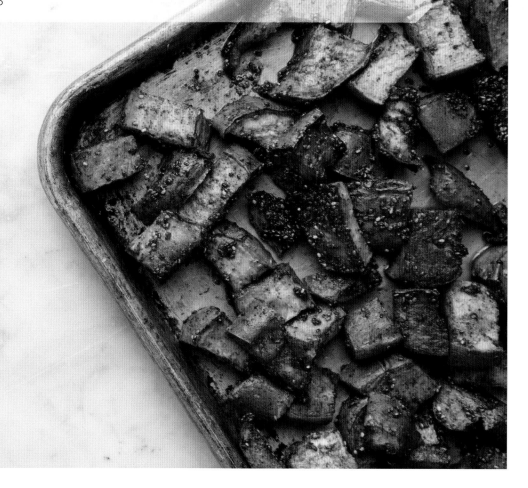

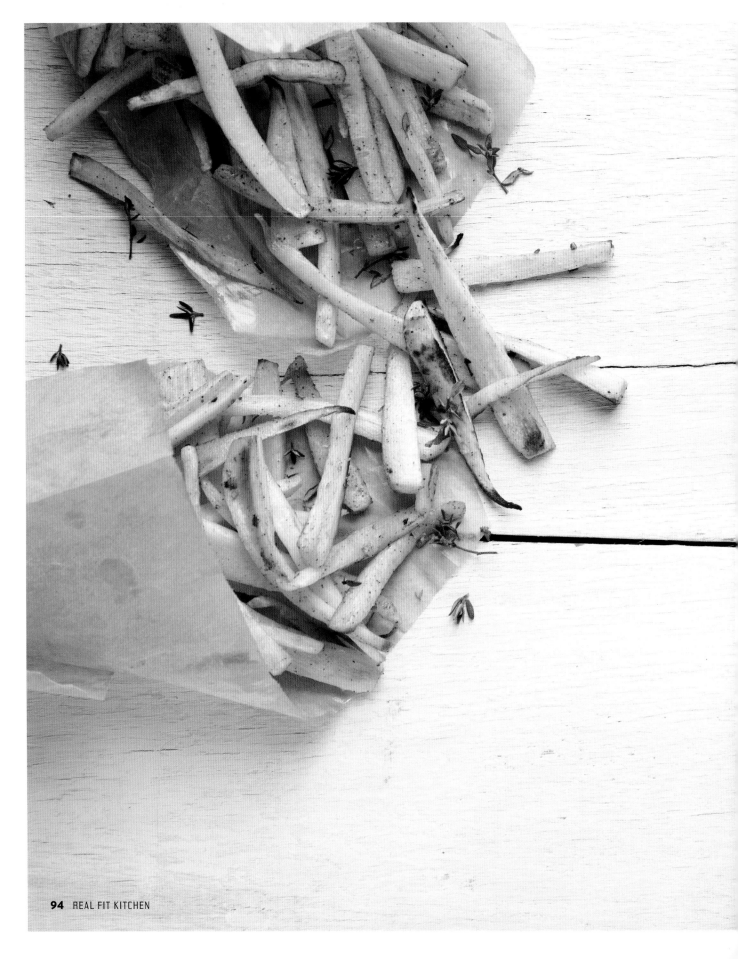

Underdog Fries

Who doesn't love a good french fry? We do, but we'll pass on the grease, the calories, and the quickly digested starch that leaves us feeling bloated. We prefer parsnip fries. These root vegetables that are often overlooked simply because of their pale appearance. These underdogs have a lightly sweet and nutty flavor and they're a great source of B vitamins, vitamin C, fiber, and the minerals iron, calcium, potassium, manganese, and phosphorus. Finally, fries you can feel good about.

2	garlic cloves, chopped or crushed (optional)
1	tablespoon (15 ml) olive oil
	Juice of 1 lemon
1	teaspoon pure maple syrup
1	teaspoon cinnamon
½	teaspoon nutmeg
1	teaspoon sea salt
½	teaspoon black pepper
4	medium parsnips, washed well, skin on
1	tablespoon (2.4 g) fresh thyme, chopped (optional)

Preheat the oven to 450°F (230°C).

Mix together the olive oil, lemon juice, maple syrup, cinnamon, nutmeg, salt, and pepper, (and garlic if you are using it) in a small bowl. Set aside.

Cut the parsnips into the size of french fries and place them in a larger bowl. Massage the olive oil mixture into the parsnip sticks, with your hands.

Roast for 30 minutes or until the outsides are light brown and the insides are tender, turning them over halfway through the cooking.

Remove from the oven, sprinkle with thyme. Let cool.

Upgrade!
This is a great replacement for **french fries, tater tots, or soft pretzels.**

Servings: 4

Notes: *Parsnips keep very well. Wrap unwashed parsnips in a paper towel and place them in a plastic or cloth storage bag. They will keep for up to 2 weeks in the refrigerator. Wash them right before you use them.*

Prefer something savory rather than sweet? Just season the parsnips with sea salt and pepper and you have fries that are just as tasty.

▶ PREWORKOUT ▶ POSTWORKOUT ▶ GLUTEN FREE ▶ DAIRY FREE ▶ VEGAN
*Low FODMAP–friendly: Omit the garlic.

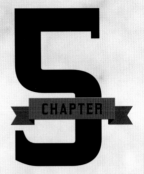

CHAPTER 5

Dressings, Dips, and Spreads

Sometimes, healthful food needs an accessory, like a room needs a punch of color from a new throw pillow. We love eating the good stuff, but sometimes we want to dress it up a bit. And the sauces and marinades in this chapter help you do just that. Learn the art of a few basic flavors and flavor combinations that will complement your food. Find a favorite and make it your own by adding your special twist. Having spices on hand, and trying new ones is the key to making your food tastier.

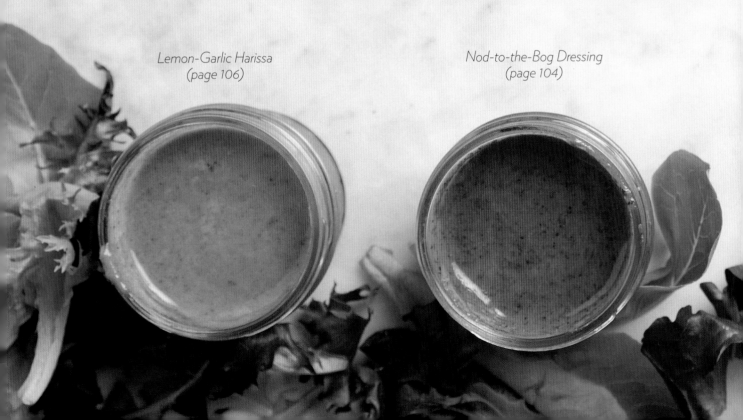

Lemon-Garlic Harissa
(page 106)

Nod-to-the-Bog Dressing
(page 104)

Edamame Citrus Spread
(page 105)

Leo's Power Pesto
(page 100)

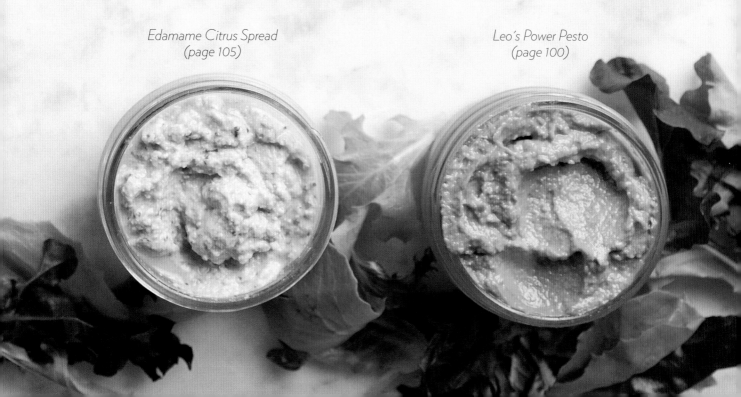

Garlic Scape Pesto

Garlic scapes are the long, spindly stalks of the garlic plant that are often tossed aside. If scapes are harvested when they are young and tender, they can be added to salads or used in sauces such as this simple pesto. The season for scapes is very short, usually late spring and early summer, so watch for them at your farmers' market. Buy as many scapes as you can and make extra pesto as a thoughtful gift for a few friends—or keep the pesto in your freezer to use on a night you are too tired to cook.

- 1 cup (160 g) coarsely chopped garlic scapes, about 5 medium-size scapes (see notes)
- ¼ cup (35 g) pine nuts
- ¼ cup (25 g) grated Parmesan or Pecorino cheese
- Juice and zest of ½ lemon
- ½ teaspoon sea salt
- ½ teaspoon black pepper
- ½ cup (120 ml) olive oil

Purée the garlic scapes, nuts, cheese, lemon juice, lemon zest, salt, and pepper in a food processor or high-performance blender until finely chopped.

With the motor running, slowly pour the oil through the top opening. Season the pesto with additional salt and pepper to taste.

Servings: 4

Notes: *The number of scapes you use here is dependent on how large the scapes are in any particular growing season.*

Fresh garlic scapes are more pungent than the frozen version and will make a stronger flavored pesto.

The pesto keeps in the refrigerator, tightly covered, for 1 week or in the freezer for about 6 months in freezer bags or ice cube trays.

Can't find garlic scapes? Substitute 1 to 2 large cloves of garlic.

▶ POSTWORKOUT ▶ NUTRIENT-PACKED MAINSTAY ▶ GLUTEN FREE ▶ LOW FODMAP

Garlic Scape~White Bean Dip

This nutrient-rich dip combines zesty garlic scapes with mild white (cannellini) beans and makes a perfect postworkout snack or a healthy party snack. Serve it with crackers, pita bread, or crudités.

½ cup (80 g) coarsely chopped garlic scapes (or substitute 1 large garlic clove)

Juice and zest of ½ lemon

½ teaspoon sea salt

½ teaspoon black pepper

1 can (15 ounces, or 400 g) cannellini beans, rinsed and drained

¼ cup (60 ml) olive oil

2 springs of fresh rosemary, coarsely chopped, for garnish (optional)

Purée the garlic scapes, lemon juice, lemon zest, salt, and pepper until finely chopped.

Add the cannellini beans and continue processing until you have a rough purée.

With the motor running, slowly pour in the olive oil into the top of the high-performance blender or food processor until the mixture is smooth. If it's too thick, pulse in a few tablespoons of water until you have the consistency of a dip.

Season with salt and pepper to taste and add more lemon juice, if you like.

Garnish with a drizzle of olive oil and fresh sprig of rosemary, or with lemon slices and a sprinkling of freshly ground black pepper.

Servings: 4

Notes: *This dip keeps in the refrigerator, tightly covered, for 1 week or in the freezer for up to 6 months.*

❱ POSTWORKOUT ❱ GLUTEN FREE ❱ DAIRY FREE ❱ VEGAN

Leo's Power Pesto

Our favorite pesto recipe comes from a Boston beekeeper, so naturally it includes honey. Light on cheese and rich with basil and arugula, this pesto has powerful antibacterial properties. The eugenol in basil's natural oils acts in a similar way to an over-the-counter anti-inflammatory medication, so ditch the pills and choose this pesto after a strenuous workout. This flavorful recipe is courtesy of Mark Lewis of The Best Bees Company. He always keeps this pesto on hand to keep his young son Leo smiling at the dinner table. Learn more about honeybees at bestbees.com.

- 2 cups (80 g) basil leaves, washed, stems trimmed
- 1 cup (20 g) arugula
- 3 cloves garlic, peeled
- ⅔ cup (155 ml) olive oil
- ½ cup (50 g) freshly grated Parmesan or Pecorino Romano, or a mixture of both
- 2 tablespoons (40 g) honey, or to taste
- 2 tablespoons (32 g) almond butter
- Sea salt and black pepper to taste

Put basil, arugula, garlic, and half the olive oil in a food processor and pulse a few times. Add the remaining olive oil and the rest of the ingredients and pulse a few more times until the ingredients are combined and the mixture is fairly smooth.

Serve on pasta, toast, or vegetables.

Servings: 8

Notes: *Whenever possible, use local honey. It tastes better, is richer in antioxidants, and is a great way to support your community.*

The pesto keeps tightly covered in the refrigerator for up to 1 week or frozen in freezer bags or in ice cube trays for up to 6 months.

Upgrade!
This recipe is a great replacement for **jarred pesto** or a **pasta sauce.**

▶ POSTWORKOUT ▶ NUTRIENT-PACKED MAINSTAY ▶ GLUTEN FREE

SSShhh (Sammy's Secret Sauce)

Sammy is our great friend, an avid cyclist, a landscape genius, and a master in the kitchen who never shares his recipes. Every year, he hosts an end-of-summer barbeque that's not to be missed. His chicken, fish, and steak are always a topic of conversation: How did he do that? Sammy's sauce taps into flavors from his native Caribbean island of Tobago, and Tara was able to create a version that's pretty close to his. This recipe will yield plenty of extra sauce—some for now, some for later.

1 yellow onion, chopped coarsely

4 green onions, chopped coarsely, white stems and rough green tops removed

2 celery stalks, leafy tops included, chopped coarsely

10 fresh thyme sprigs, washed well, stems included

4 garlic cloves, peeled

1 tablespoon (9 g) seeded and chopped hot pepper (red jalapeño or small Fresno chili)

2 cups (120 g) fresh Italian parsley (about half a bunch, stems included), washed well

2 tablespoons (30 ml) reduced-sodium tamari sauce (gluten-free soy sauce)

2 tablespoons (30 ml) white or red vinegar

½ teaspoon sea salt

½ teaspoon black pepper

2 ounces (60 ml) water

Wash the fresh ingredients well. Chop the onion, green onions, and celery and put them in the blender.

Add the thyme sprigs, garlic cloves, hot pepper, parsley, tamari sauce, vinegar, salt, and pepper to the blender. Add the water.

Blend on high speed until smooth. Add more water, if necessary until the marinade is fairly thick but smooth and uniform.

Use the sauce on chicken breasts and thighs, steak, fish, or vegetables.

Servings: 4 to 6 (enough sauce to cover about 6 large chicken breasts)

Notes: *Sammy recommends marinating the chicken breasts in a freezer bag. Make sure the marinade covers the breasts well and keep them in the refrigerator overnight. When you're ready to cook, remove the chicken and put it in a baking pan. Cover with foil and bake for 30 minutes at 350°F (180°C). Carefully remove the foil and continue to bake for another 15 minutes.*

If you are using the sauce with fish, tofu, or tempeh, marinate for 1 to 2 hours. Grill or bake as you would with your favorite protein.

This sauce keeps, tightly sealed, for up to 1 week in the refrigerator or for 3 months in the freezer.

Upgrade!
This is a great replacement for **bottled marinades.**

▶ GLUTEN FREE ▶ DAIRY FREE ▶ VEGAN

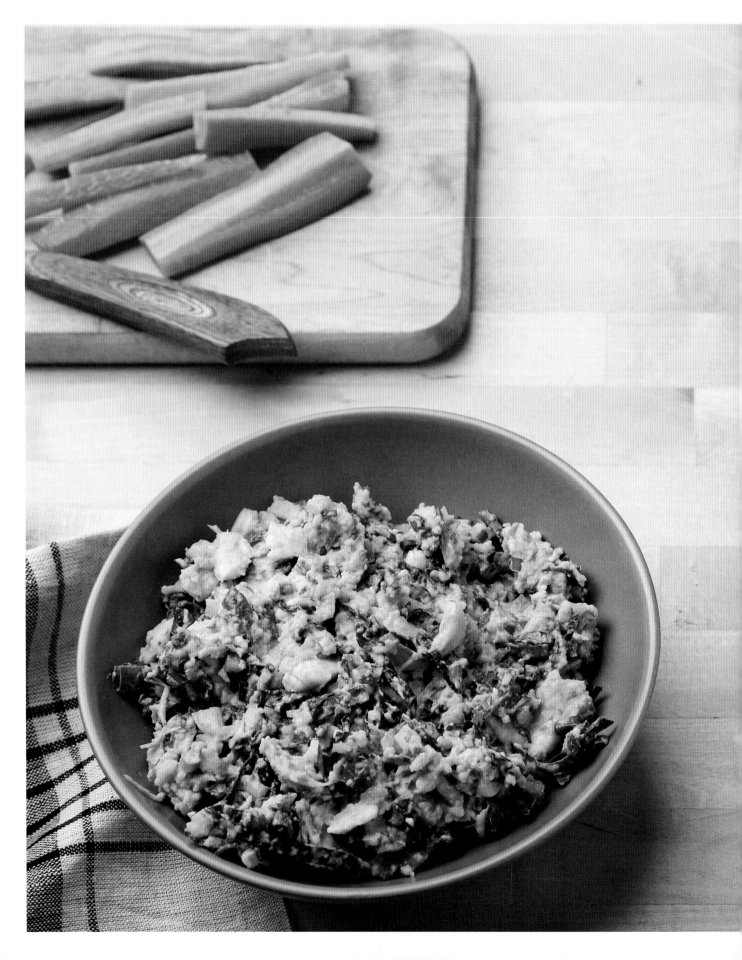

Guac~Kale~Mole

What better way to supercharge guacamole than by adding kale? We asked the kale expert herself, Elise from Kale and Chocolate, to give us her perfect recipe. More of her recipes can be found at kaleandchocolate.com.

2 to 3 avocados

Juice of 1 lime

¼ cup (40 g) red onion, chopped

½ clove garlic, chopped

½ jalapeño pepper, chopped

2 tablespoons (2 g) cilantro

¼ teaspoon cumin

4 to 5 large kale leaves, stems and stalk removed, finely chopped

Mix together all the ingredients, except for the kale.

Stir in the finely chopped kale.

Serve with chips or with sticks of jicama, carrots, red pepper, or use in a salad.

Servings: 6

Notes: *If you have a prepared guacamole that you love, add the kale to it. Make sure you massage the kale with some olive oil to soften it before you mix it in.*

Upgrade!
This recipe is a great replacement for **traditional guacamole** or **creamy dips.**

DID YOU KNOW? **Kale is high in iron, vitamin K, antioxidants, vitamin A, vitamin C, and calcium. As you train hard, you need more vitamins and minerals to keep you healthy, and help to repair your muscles. Adding more kale to your diet is a fantastic way to take your game to the next level. The more, the better!**

▶ GLUTEN FREE ▶ DAIRY FREE ▶ VEGAN

Nod~to~the~Bog Dressing

We call New England home and, naturally, love our fresh cranberries. They are full of vitamin C and other health-promoting phytonutrients. Studies of their antioxidant, anti-inflammatory, and anticancer properties confirm the impressive benefits of eating the whole berry, not the highly processed juice or the sugary dried ones. Whole cranberries are available frozen all year. This tart dressing will add a pop of color and a blast of nutrients to your favorite salad.

¼ cup (25 g) fresh or frozen cranberries

1 tablespoon (11 g) Dijon mustard

1 garlic clove, peeled

1 tablespoon (15 ml) apple cider vinegar (preferably organic, raw, unpasteurized, and unfiltered)

2 tablespoons (40 g) local honey (or pure maple syrup)

2 tablespoons (30 ml) extra-virgin olive oil

¼ cup (60 ml) water

½ teaspoon sea salt

¼ teaspoon black pepper

Rinse the cranberries well and put them in blender. Add the remaining ingredients.

Blend on high speed until smooth. Add more water, if necessary, so the dressing is smooth. Add more salt and pepper to taste.

Use this dressing on your favorite salad, massaging it gently into the greens. Or serve it in a bowl or pitcher to dress the salad individually.

Servings: 4

Notes: *This recipe can also be used as a marinade for chicken breasts or tempeh.*

This dressing keeps, tightly sealed, for up to 1 week in the refrigerator or for 1 month in the freezer.

❯ GLUTEN FREE ❯ DAIRY FREE ❯ VEGAN
*Low FODMAP–friendly: Omit the garlic or use garlic-infused oil. **Vegan: Use pure maple syrup instead of honey.

Edamame Citrus Spread

Edamame are boiled, young soy beans. They are usually eaten as a snack or added to a salad or side dish. This recipe yields a smooth nutty spread that's loaded with fiber, protein, healthy fat, and vitamins. Edamame can be found in the frozen food area of the grocery store.

2 cups (260 g) frozen shelled edamame

pinch sea salt

3 garlic cloves, peeled

½ cup (20 g) fresh basil leaves (or mint), tightly packed

2 tablespoons (18 g) pine nuts (toasted, see notes)

2 tablespoons (30 g) plain Greek yogurt

2 tablespoons (22 g) Dijon mustard

2 tablespoons (30 ml) olive oil

2 tablespoons (10 ml) fresh lemon juice

1 teaspoon hot sauce (optional)

Zest of 1 lemon

¼ cup (60 ml) water

Sea salt and black pepper to taste

Fill a small saucepan about halfway with water. Add a pinch of salt and bring to a boil.

Cook the edamame for about 5 minutes or until tender. Remove the pan from the heat and drain the edamame in a strainer. Combine the edamame, garlic, basil, pine nuts, yogurt, and mustard in a food processor or high performance blender. Pulse the mixture about 7 to 10 times or until coarsely ground. Add the remaining ingredients and process until nearly smooth.

Serve this spread with mini toasts, crackers, or on top of lettuce cups.

Servings: 8 ¼-cup (56 g) servings

Notes: *Toasted pine nuts add a slightly smoky flavor to this recipe. To toast them, place the pine nuts in a naked pan (no salt, no pepper, no oil) on medium heat for 2 minutes, tossing them every 30 seconds until they start to brown slightly. Remove them from the heat and allow them to cool. Watch them carefully or you will burn them (we certainly have, multiple times). Consider it a mindfulness exercise—be here now.*

Upgrade!
This is a great replacement for **creamy spreads and dips.**

▶ GLUTEN FREE

Halftime Hummus

Chickpeas, the main ingredient in hummus, are rich in fiber, protein, iron, and will help you feel satisfied longer. This hummus makes a quick snack and is great with cut-up vegetables after a workout.

2 cups (430 g) cooked or 1 can (16 ounces, or 448 g) chickpeas
2 garlic cloves, chopped
⅓ cup (80 g) tahini
¼ cup (60 ml) olive oil
¼ cup (60 ml) hot water
Juice of 2 lemons
1½ teaspoons sea salt

Blend all ingredients in a food processor or high-performance blender.

Serve in a bowl with crackers or crudité for dipping.

Servings: 10 ¼-cup (56 g) servings

Notes: *You can easily add flavor to hummus by adding ingredients like roasted red pepper, jalapeño pepper, or cilantro.*

Can't find tahini? Leave it out. Add more lemon juice or a little water if you desire, to make it a thinner consistency.

Upgrade!
Store-bought hummus typically uses inexpensive oils for mass production. This homemade version is an automatic upgrade, and we think you'll taste the difference, too.

▶ POSTWORKOUT ▶ GLUTEN FREE ▶ DAIRY FREE ▶ VEGAN

Lemon~Garlic Harissa

Here is a tangy marinade, dip, spread, and dressing, all in one.

¼ cup (60 ml) olive oil
¼ cup (85 g) honey or pure maple syrup
Juice of 2 lemons
Zest of 1 lemon
½ large shallot, crushed
4 large garlic cloves, crushed
½ tablespoon Hungarian paprika
1½ teaspoons harissa
1 tablespoon (15 ml) distilled white vinegar
1 teaspoon sea salt
1 teaspoon black pepper

Mix ingredients together with a whisk or in a blender.

When using this sauce for chicken breasts, steak or tempeh, marinate the protein at least 4 hours or overnight, and marinate fish for 1 to 2 hours.

Servings: 4 (covers about 4 to 6 chicken breasts)

Note: *Make extra sauce and store it in small mason jars in the refrigerator and you will always have extra flavor on hand.*

Upgrade!
This is a great replacement for **commercial sauces** and **marinades** that are loaded with excess sugar and preservatives.

▶ GLUTEN FREE ▶ DAIRY FREE
*Vegan: Use pure maple syrup.

Carrot Cake Nut Butter

Have some vegetables in your nut butter. Yes! We love carrot cake nut butter because it supercharges your nut butter with the nutritional benefits of carrots. It is perfect to spread on a banana, figs, brown rice tortillas, or sprouted grain toast.

- 2 cups (275 g) raw cashews or almonds
- 1 cup (130 g) chopped carrots
- 2 teaspoons (5 g) maca powder
- 2 teaspoons (5 g) cinnamon
- ½ teaspoon sea salt
- 1 teaspoon vanilla extract

Blend all ingredients together in a high-performance blender or a food processor until smooth and creamy.

Store the nut butter in a mason jar in the refrigerator for up to 1 month.

Servings: 24

Notes: It is easy to overdo it on the nut butter. Two tablespoons turns into four, very quickly. Try freezing the nut butter into premade serving sizes in ice cube trays. It makes it harder to dip your spoon in a few too many times.

Upgrade!
This is a great replacement for **store-bought peanut butter.** It also makes a great gift for your favorite athlete.

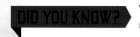 **DID YOU KNOW?** We all know that carrots protect our eyes, but did you know their high antioxidant content also may help protect our arteries from inflammation?

▶ POSTWORKOUT ▶ GLUTEN FREE ▶ DAIRY FREE ▶ VEGAN
*Low FODMAP–friendly: Use almonds instead of cashews.

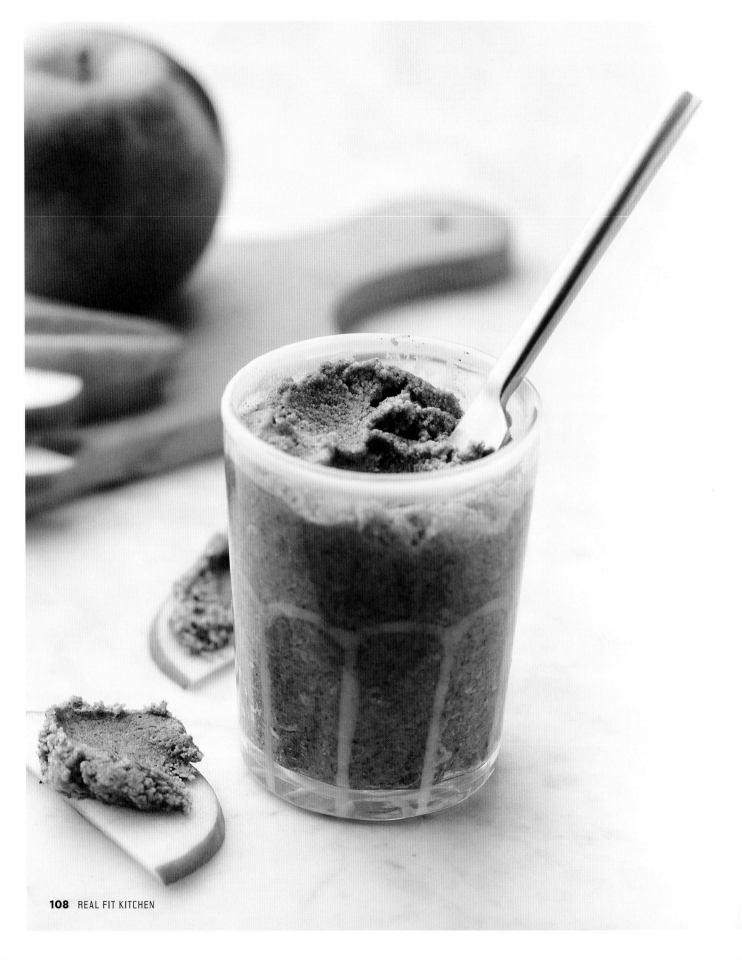

Cinnamon Pecan Nut Butter

We like to change up our nut butter—we usually boost it with maca, a powerful ingredient that helps the body respond better to stress. Cinnamon adds a sweet flavor without using sugar and offers powerful anti-inflammatory and antimicrobial benefits.

2 cups (200 g) raw pecans

1 cup (135 g) raw cashews

2 teaspoons (5 g) maca powder

1 teaspoon cinnamon

½ teaspoon sea salt

Blend all the ingredients together in a high performance blender or a food processor until the mixture is smooth and creamy.

Servings: 24

Note: *We often carry our own nut butters in portable mini mason jars. See cuppow.com for a range of options.*

❱ POSTWORKOUT ❱ GLUTEN FREE ❱ DAIRY FREE ❱ VEGAN
*Low FODMAP–friendly: Replace the cashews with almonds.

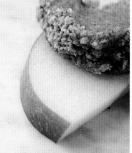

Champion Chocolate Hazelnut Spread

We get asked about chocolate-hazelnut spreads all the time because they are often marketed as healthy for athletes. Our version boasts all the chocolate-hazelnut goodness you need to fuel your body and nothing you don't.

1¼ cup (35 g) raw hazelnuts

½ cup (43 g) raw cacao powder

¾ cup (180 g) chickpeas, cooked or canned

⅓ cup (107 g) pure maple syrup

1 tablespoon (14 g) coconut oil

1 tablespoon (15 ml) vanilla extract

1 tablespoon (15 ml) coconut milk

½ teaspoon sea salt

Preheat the oven to 350°F (180°C).

Place the hazelnuts on a baking sheet and roast them for 15 minutes.

Combine the roasted hazelnuts and the remaining ingredients in a high-performance blender or food processor and process until smooth.

Servings: 8

Notes: If you have a high-speed blender with a plunger, use medium speed and plunge the ingredients until smooth. If you want a smoother spread, slowly add more coconut milk, being careful not to add too much.

Upgrade!
Store-bought chocolate spreads are full of unhealthy and highly processed ingredients such as sugar, palm oil, and stabilizers just to give them a longer shelf life.

DID YOU KNOW? Hazelnuts are an excellent source of folate and a good source of vitamin E. It's best to get vitamin E from food rather than from supplements. Some research suggests that the synthetic vitamin form may even hamper endurance performance.

▶ POSTWORKOUT ▶ NUTRIENT-PACKED TREAT ▶ GLUTEN FREE ▶ DAIRY FREE ▶ VEGAN
▶ LOW FODMAP

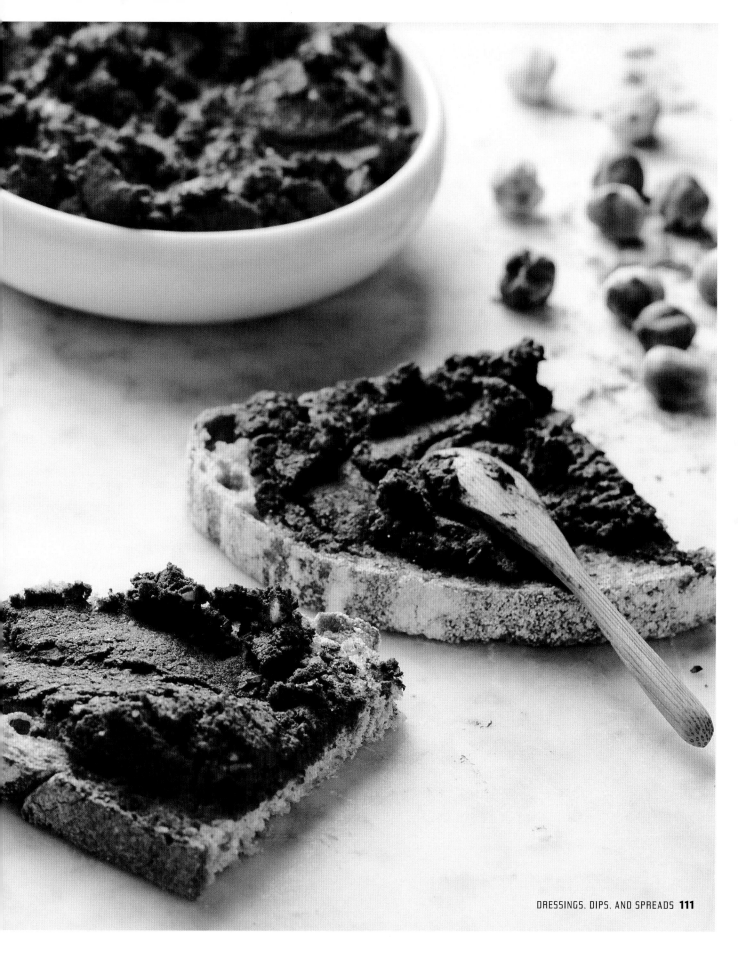

Mellow Mallow

If you grew up in the northeastern United States, you very likely ate Fluffernutter sandwiches (peanut butter and marshmallow creme) as a kid. After a fund-raising bike ride where they served peanut butter and marshmallow creme sandwiches as fuel at the rest stops, we were inspired to create a healthier version (without the corn syrup) of our favorite childhood spread. Russ and Shari are the husband-and-wife team behind Apotheker's, maker of handcrafted chocolate, marsh-mallows, and confections using ethically sourced ingredients. They re-created a childhood favorite here. Visit them at apothekerskitchen.com.

1 cup (322 g) pure maple syrup

1 egg white

1½ teaspoons vanilla extract

Place the egg white in the bowl of an electric mixer and start beating on medium speed.

While egg white is beating, heat the maple syrup until it comes to a light boil.

When egg white is firm and fluffy, slowly add the heated maple syrup to it while continuing to beat. Mix in a small amount of syrup at a time and wait until it is completely incorporated before adding more.

When all maple syrup has been incorporated, add the vanilla extract.

Continue mixing on medium speed for about 5 minutes or until the mixture has become lighter and is fluffy.

Store the mixture in the refrigerator for up to 1 week.

Servings: 4

Upgrade!
This recipe is a great replacement for **jarred marshmallow creme.**

DID YOU KNOW? Maple syrup contains B vitamins, manganese, calcium, iron, zinc, polyphenols, and antioxidant compounds. Like any sweetener, it should be used sparingly. But, when choosing a sweetener, pure maple syrup is our natural favorite.

▶ NUTRIENT-PACKED TREAT ▶ GLUTEN FREE ▶ DAIRY FREE

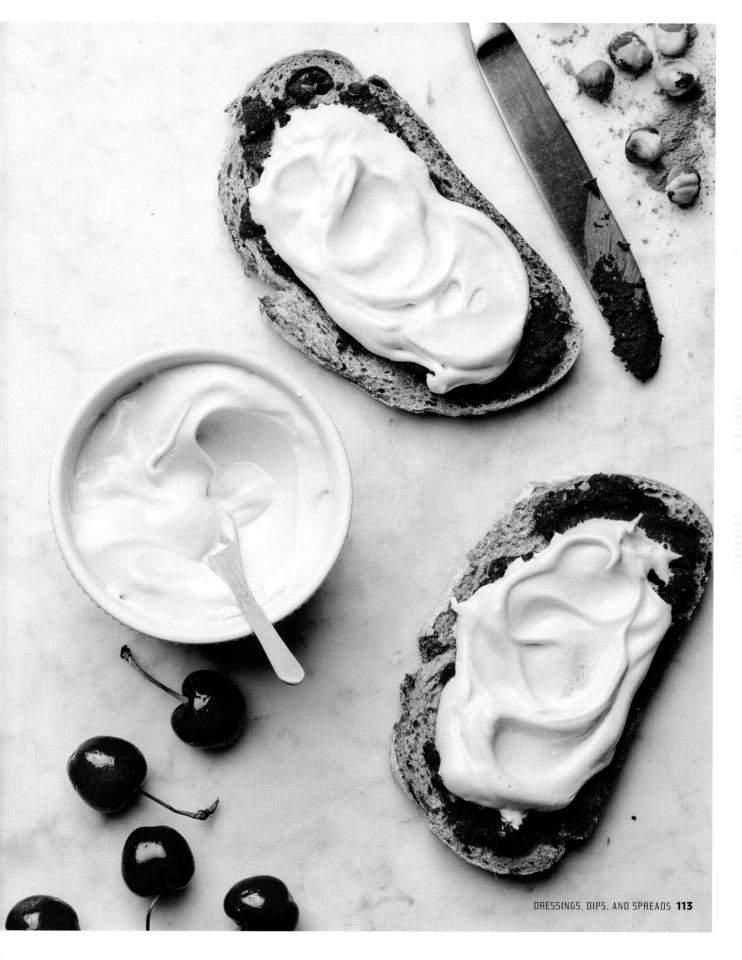

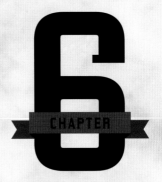

6

CHAPTER

Desserts

We probably could have created an entire cookbook of desserts. We believe healthy eating and consistent exercise provides ample wiggle room to include an occasional decadent treat. Our desserts avoid the processed white sugar found in many commercial products. The recipes in this chapter are natural, guilt free, and help satisfy your sweet tooth. A deliciously good dessert, in a small amount is the perfect way to end the day!

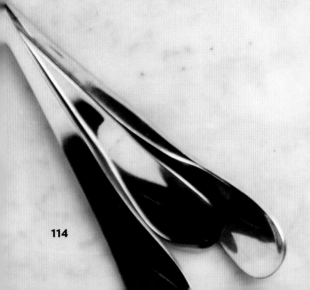

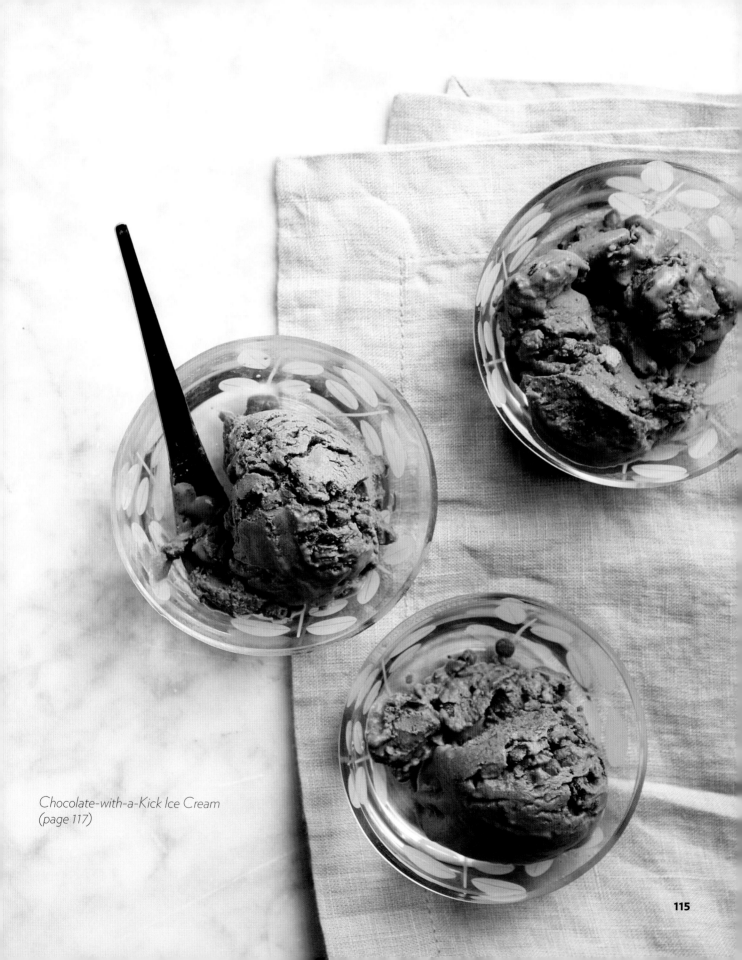

Chocolate-with-a-Kick Ice Cream
(page 117)

Vanilla~Cacao Nib Ice Cream

Katelyn Williams of Scoop Sights started making dairy-free ice cream in her home and we were lucky enough to be a part of the early taste testing. Katelyn is an ice cream connoisseur, but as an avid runner and yogi, she wanted to create a healthier treat. This is her twist on classic chocolate chip ice cream. She now sells pints and pops, too; check out her site scoopsights.com.

2 cans (12 ounces, or 355 g each) full-fat organic coconut milk

2 vanilla beans

¼ to ½ cup (60 to 115 g) coconut sugar (according to taste)

2 tablespoons (11 g) raw cacao powder

1 teaspoon maca powder

1 teaspoon vanilla

pinch sea salt

¼ cup (44 g) raw cacao nibs

Pour off the coconut milk into a jar and set aside to use another time. Scrape out the coconut cream that has settled at the bottom of the can into a pot and heat over medium heat.

Scrape out the seeds from the center of the vanilla beans and add both seeds and pods to the coconut cream, stirring until the coconut cream is melted. Allow the mixture to sit for 1 hour over low heat.

Remove the vanilla beans and add the coconut sugar, cacao powder, maca powder, vanilla, and salt. Stir until thoroughly mixed.

Strain this mixture through a fine-mesh strainer and refrigerate for about 2 hours or until cold. You want the mixture to be very cold when you put it into the ice cream maker to decrease the chance of ice crystals forming.

Freeze according to your ice cream maker's instructions. Add the cacao nibs into the ice cream maker when it is churning. Transfer the mixture to the freezer for 1 hour for harder ice cream, or enjoy the soft creamy ice cream immediately.

Servings: 4

Upgrade! Traditional ice cream is full of low-quality dairy and sugar. Why not give a favorite treat a simple nutrition makeover?

▶ NUTRIENT-PACKED TREAT ▶ GLUTEN FREE ▶ DAIRY FREE ▶ VEGAN

Chocolate~with~a~Kick Ice Cream

This recipe is also from Katelyn Williams of Scoop Sights and the flavor was inspired by her need for something chocolate, but with a kick. Being from New Orleans, she likes to spice up everything, including her desserts. You can find her at scoopsights.com.

- 2 cups (455 ml) full-fat coconut milk
- 6 dates or ¼ cup (60 g) coconut sugar
- ½ cup (87 g) dairy-free chocolate chips
- 1 teaspoon cayenne
- 2 teaspoons (5 g) cinnamon
- 1 teaspoon vanilla
- pinch sea salt

Put the coconut cream and dates (or coconut sugar) in a high performance blender and blend until smooth.

In a saucepan over medium-low heat, melt the chocolate chips, and add the cinnamon and cayenne.

Pour the melted chocolate mixture into the coconut cream base and blend.

Add the vanilla and salt, blend, and refrigerate the mixture.

Churn the mixture according to your ice cream maker's instructions.

Top the ice cream with fresh cinnamon.

Servings: 4

Notes: *After you add the cinnamon and cayenne to the melting chocolate, you can taste it—carefully since it will be hot—and add extra cinnamon or, as Katelyn likes it, extra cayenne!*

▸ NUTRIENT-PACKED TREAT ▸ GLUTEN FREE ▸ DAIRY FREE ▸ VEGAN

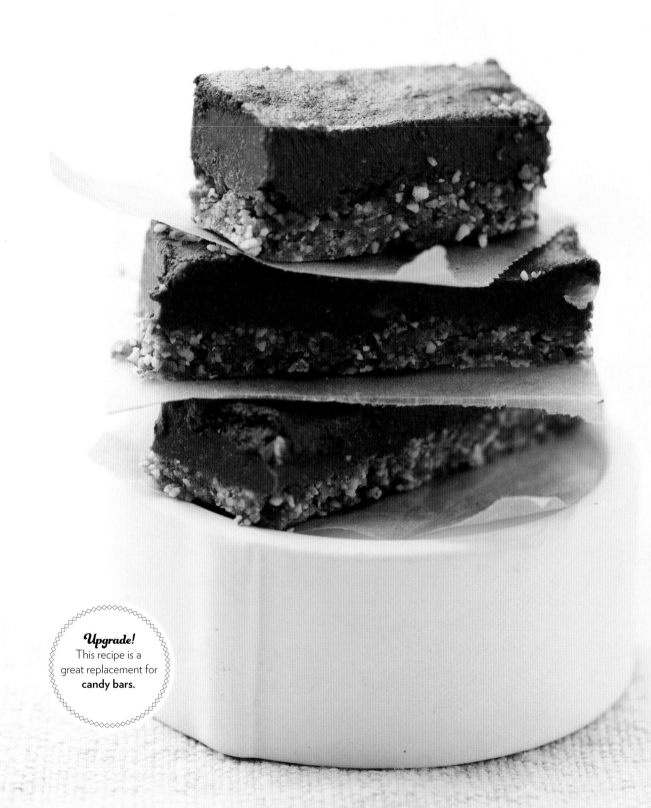

Upgrade!
This recipe is a great replacement for **candy bars.**

Raw Coconut~Caramel Cream Bars

These bars are straight from the kitchen of Charlotte of kaleyeahcatering.com. These tasty little bars are a much healthier version than a candy bar when you are looking for a sweet treat.

Crust:

- 1 cup (145 g) raw almonds
- 1 cup (178 g) dates, pitted
  pinch sea salt

Caramel:

- ½ cup (130 g) cashew butter
- ½ cup (109 g) unrefined coconut oil
- 3 tablespoons (16 g) cacao powder
- ¼ cup (80 g) pure maple syrup
- 1 teaspoon vanilla

Chocolate Cream:

- ⅓ cup (73 g) coconut oil
- 3 tablespoons (16 g) cacao powder
- ¼ cup (80 g) pure maple syrup
- 1 teaspoon vanilla

To make the crust, process the almonds into flour in a food processor or high-performance blender.

Add the dates and pulse until the dough comes together.

Press the dough into the bottom of a parchment paper–lined 8-inch (20 cm) square baking pan and refrigerate.

To make the caramel, combine all the ingredients in a blender. Spread the caramel on top of the crust.

To make the chocolate cream, blend all the ingredients together. Spread the cream on top of the caramel.

Servings: 6

Notes: *We prefer Medjool dates because they are softer and easier to work with. Make sure you remove the pits!*

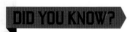 **DID YOU KNOW?** **Dates are nature's candy. They have quite a bit of sugar, but are loaded with minerals like iron, manganese, and magnesium.**

Raw cacao is the raw form of cacao beans before they are processed into chocolate. Cacao is loaded with antioxidants and polyphenols, which can help reduce inflammation and is more nutrient rich than cocoa powder. Raw cacao is also a good source of iron and magnesium, minerals that help with proper muscle function.

▶ NUTRIENT-PACKED TREAT ▶ GLUTEN FREE ▶ DAIRY FREE ▶ VEGAN

Biked Apples

On a sunny fall Saturday, Tara and some friends biked from Boston to Honey Pot Hill Orchards. Waiting patiently to pay to pick apples but hungry from the hilly 35-mile (56 km) ride, they took a detour to Honey Pot's farm store and bought a fresh apple pie, hot from the oven. They sat down on a few hay bales and devoured the pie (with no forks or knives). With very sticky fingers, they picked apples and then biked back to Boston with their heavy load. The memory of that day inspired this healthier version of an apple dessert that Kate and her triathlon training partner and DRINKmaple business partner Jeff now describe as a favorite postworkout treat after long bike rides.

4	apples, cored, skin on
2	tablespoons (32 g) almond butter
2	tablespoons (40 g) pure maple syrup
1	teaspoon cinnamon
¼	cup (28 g) pecans or walnuts, chopped
¼	cup (28 g) cranberries, fresh or dried
⅛	teaspoon ground cloves
	pinch sea salt

Preheat the oven to 375°F (190°C) and core the apples.

Combine the almond butter, maple syrup, cinnamon, nuts, cranberries, cloves, and salt in a bowl and mix together.

Place the mixture in the core of each apple, dividing it evenly.

Bake for 30 minutes.

Serve the apples with a fork and knife.

Servings: 4

Notes: *An apple corer is very helpful gadget for this recipe. If you don't have one, you can improvise by cutting the apples into quarters and adding the mixture on top to create more of an apple crisp.*

Upgrade!
This recipe is a great replacement for **apple pie** or **apple crisp.**

DID YOU KNOW? Cloves contain eugenol, an anti-inflammatory. Cloves may also aid in digestion.

▶ POSTWORKOUT ▶ NUTRIENT-PACKED TREAT ▶ GLUTEN FREE ▶ DAIRY FREE ▶ VEGAN

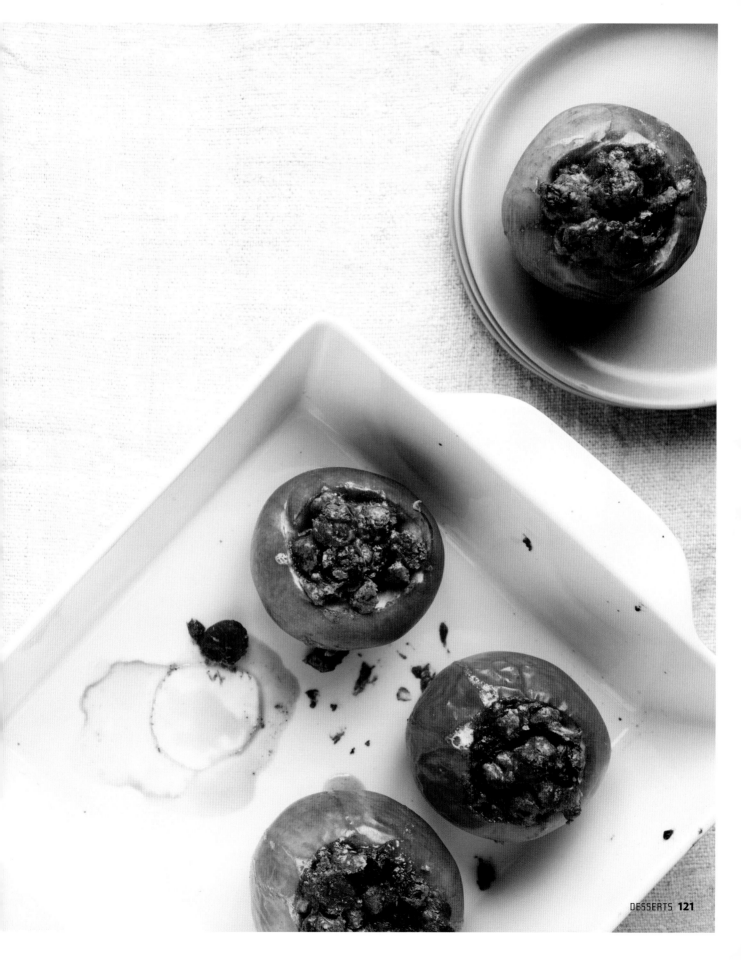

Beantown Brownies

We do not believe in "cheat meals" or "cheat foods." We do believe in giving homemade sweets an upgrade. Sneak some fiber into your desserts, and you will find that you're satisfied with a smaller portion. These brownies get a nutrient boost from the black beans, but you notice only the taste of the rich chocolate.

- 1 can (14 ounces, or 396 g) black beans, rinsed and drained
- 3 pitted prunes
- 1½ cups (260 g) dark chocolate bark or squares (70% cacao solids), melted
- 3 large eggs
- ½ cup (120 g) avocado about half a medium avocado

- 4 tablespoons (56 g) coconut or avocado oil
- ⅔ cup (230 g) honey
- ⅔ cup (82 g) all-purpose flour
- 3 tablespoons (16 g) raw cacao powder
- 2 teaspoons (10 ml) vanilla extract
- Zest of 2 lemons

- 1 teaspoon Aleppo chili flakes (optional)
- 2 teaspoons (9 g) baking powder
- ½ teaspoon baking soda
- 3 tablespoons (30 ml) whole milk
- 2 tablespoons (23 g) cacao nibs for topping (optional)

Preheat the oven to 325°F (170°C).

Grease a 10-inch (25 cm) square baking pan and line it with parchment paper.

Place the beans and prunes in a food processor or high-performance blender and grind them into a crumbly paste.

Add the melted chocolate, eggs, avocado, and oil, and process until smooth.

Add the honey, flour, cacao powder, vanilla, lemon zest, chili flakes (if desired), baking powder, and baking soda. Process until blended together.

Add the milk.

Pour the brownie mixture into the prepared pan and level it with a spatula. Sprinkle cacao nibs on top if desired.

Bake for about 20 minutes or until the top is crisp and the edges are curling away from the pan slightly. Allow the brownies to cool, and then cut into 12 squares.

Upgrade!
This recipe is a great replacement for **brownies, cake,** or **cookies**.

Servings: 12

Notes: Try toppings like ½ cup (80 g) dried cherries or currants; or dust brownies with powdered sugar, extra lemon zest, and mint to garnish.

❯ POSTWORKOUT ❯ NUTRIENT-PACKED TREAT
*Gluten free: Use gluten-free, all-purpose flour. **Dairy free: Use full-fat coconut milk.

First Place Pudding

We knew this pudding was good when it tricked vegetable haters into eating spinach! This is an indulgence, but it's a great way to sneak more nutrition into your dessert.

- 2 avocados
- ⅔ cup (230 g) raw honey or pure maple syrup
- ½ cup (43 g) raw cacao powder
- 2 handfuls baby spinach
- 1 teaspoon of grass-fed gelatin (optional)

Blend all ingredients into a high performance blender or food processor until smooth.

Put the mixture in a bowl and refrigerate for 20 minutes.

Servings: 4

Notes: *Gelatin isn't necessary for the recipe, but it adds natural collagen and glucosomine to the dessert—good for the digestive tract, joint health, skin, hair, and nails.*

▶ POSTWORKOUT ▶ NUTRIENT-PACKED TREAT ▶ GLUTEN FREE ▶ DAIRY FREE
*Vegan: Leave out the gelatin.

Berry Easy Ice Cream

This is a simple, no frills "ice cream" that you can make in a blender. It is not as stable as regular ice cream, but you do not need an ice cream maker.

- 2½ cup (375 g) frozen blueberries, strawberries, or raspberries
- 1 frozen banana
- 2 tablespoons (22 g) chia seeds
- 1 teaspoon vanilla extract
- 1 tablespoon (15 g) each cacao nibs and coconut for topping (optional)

Put all ingredients except the toppings in a high-performance blender or food processor and blend until smooth.

Serve immediately.

Servings: 2

Notes: *We like the natural sweetness of the fruit, but if you like your ice cream sweeter, you can add some raw honey, pure maple syrup, or Medjool dates to taste. If the mixture is too thick, slowly add some water while blending.*

Upgrade!
This recipe is a great replacement for **ice cream** or **sorbet.**

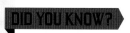 **DID YOU KNOW?** One of the highest antioxidant-rich foods readily available, blueberries are potent protectors of the heart, the mind, and the body. We don't need to tell you how delicious they are!

▶ PREWORKOUT ▶ POSTWORKOUT ▶ GLUTEN FREE ▶ DAIRY FREE ▶ VEGAN

EJ's Pumpkin Chia Seed Pudding

Elizabeth Jarrard is a dietitian in Denver where she works as a content specialist at Vega, a leader in plant-based nutrition products. She is passionate about helping people eat in a healthier and more sustainable way, and she leads by example. While we miss her energy at our intense November Project workouts in Boston, she's part of the November Project tribe in Denver. We feel her love of good food through her Instagram, @elizabetheats. Her chia pudding recipe, a snack rich in plant-based omega-3 fatty acids, is easy to make.

1	cup (250 ml) unsweetened vanilla almond milk
⅓	cup (50 g) chia seeds
⅓	cup (80 g) puréed pumpkin
1	teaspoon pure maple syrup
¼	teaspoon vanilla extract
	Sea salt, cinnamon, nutmeg, and ground cloves to taste

Mix all the ingredients (except chia seeds) together in a bowl. Gradually mix in the chia seeds 1 tablespoon (11 g) at a time. Allow the mixture to sit in the refrigerator for a minimum of 4 hours or overnight.

Enjoy as a snack or dessert or even for breakfast!

Servings: 1 ½-cup (180 g) serving or 2 ¾-cup (90 g) servings

Upgrade!
This recipe is a great replacement for **traditional pudding** or **oatmeal.**

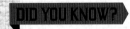
DID YOU KNOW? Chia seeds, unlike flaxseeds, do not have to be ground first for better absorption of nutrients. The seeds are rich in omega-3 fatty acids, protein, and antioxidants.

❱ PREWORKOUT ❱ POSTWORKOUT ❱ NUTRIENT-PACKED MAINSTAY
❱ NUTRIENT-PACKED TREAT ❱ GLUTEN FREE ❱ DAIRY FREE ❱ VEGAN

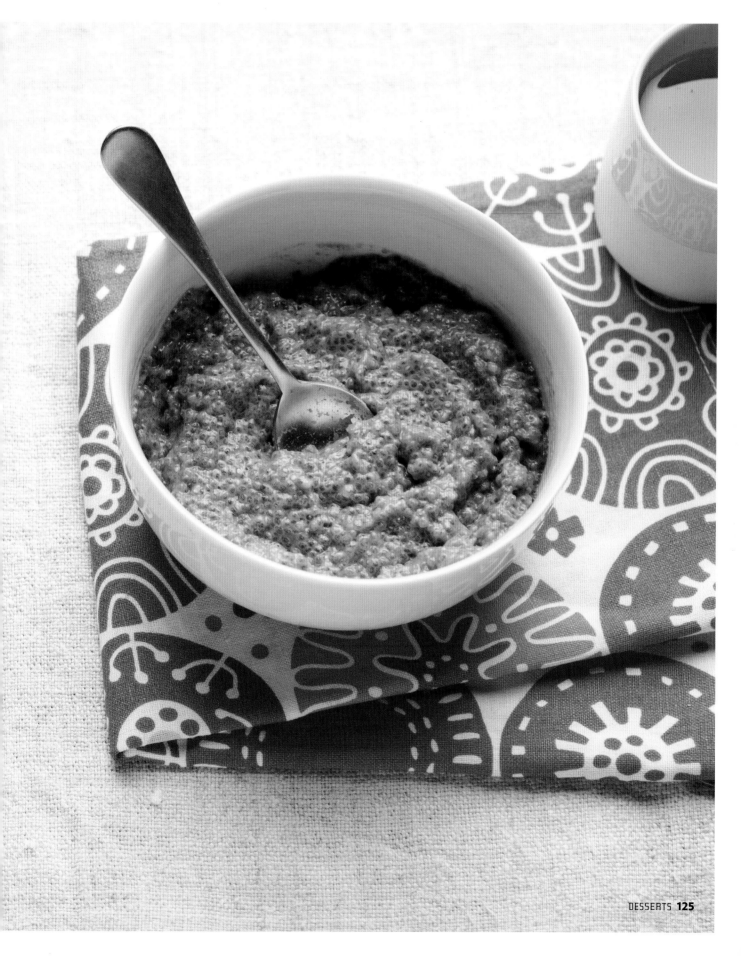

HeartBeet Cupcakes

We love to find ways to sneak more beets into our meals, fresh juices, and even into our desserts. You won't even know that this superfood root vegetable is hiding in these delicious chocolate cupcakes.

For the cupcakes:
- 1 cup (250 ml) water
- 1 cup (100 g) brown rice flour
- ¾ cup (241 g) pure maple syrup
- 1 cup (86 g) cacao powder
- 1 cup raw beets (about 1 large beet)
- ⅔ cup (150 g) grass-fed butter or coconut oil
- ⅓ cup (80 ml) coconut milk
- 4 eggs
- 1 ½ teaspoons baking powder
- ½ teaspoon sea salt
- 1 teaspoon vanilla

For the frosting:
- ¼ cup (56 g) grass-fed butter
- ¼ cup (54 g) coconut oil
- 2 tablespoons (40 g) raw honey
- 1 teaspoon vanilla
- 3 tablespoons (26 g) cashews, chopped
- ½ teaspoon lemon juice

Preheat oven to 350°F (180°C).

Line a muffin tin with 6 cupcake liners.

Combine all ingredients for the cupcakes in a high performance blender and blend until smooth.

Pour the mixture into the prepared pan and bake for 30 minutes.

For the frosting, combine all the ingredients in a food processor or high-performance blender and blend until smooth.

Allow the cupcakes to cool for 15 minutes before frosting them.

Servings: 12 muffins

Notes: *If you do not have a high-performance blender, you may want to boil the beets for 15 minutes to soften them. The cupcakes will stay fresh for a couple of days. Keep some of them in the freezer if you don't plan to eat them right away.*

Upgrade!
This recipe is a great replacement for **cupcakes, muffins, doughnuts,** or **cookies.**

▶ PREWORKOUT ▶ POSTWORKOUT ▶ NUTRIENT-PACKED TREAT ▶ GLUTEN FREE ▶ DAIRY FREE

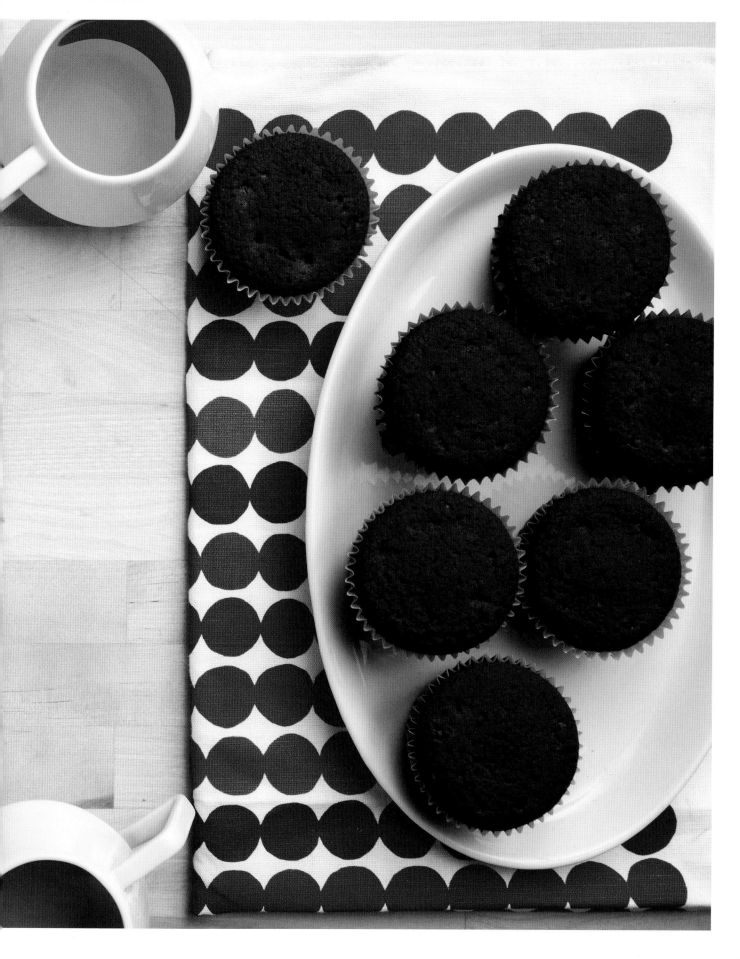

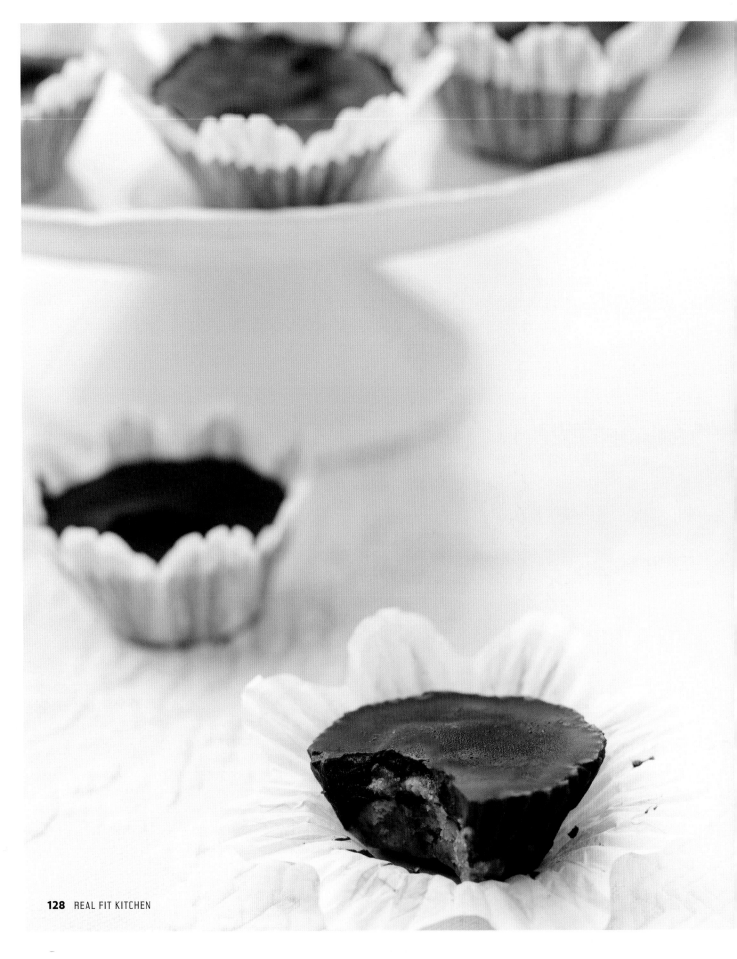

Almond Butter Cups

We shamelessly tried to convince our editor that healthy can also be tasty. We used these almond butter cups to prove it. It worked.

For the filling:

- 4 tablespoons (64 g) unsweetened almond butter
- 2 tablespoons (40 g) pure maple syrup

For the chocolate topping:

- ⅓ cup (74 g) coconut oil
- ⅓ cup (29 g) raw cacao powder
- 2 tablespoons (40 g) pure maple syrup
- ½ teaspoon vanilla extract
- ½ teaspoon sea salt

Line 8 mini or 4 standard-size muffin tins with muffin liners.

In a bowl, mix together the almond butter and the maple syrup for the filling.

In a small saucepan, heat the coconut oil on very low heat.

Add the cacao powder, maple syrup, vanilla extract, and salt to the oil and mix until smooth. Remove from the heat. Place the almond butter filling in each liner. Pour the chocolate topping over the filling.

Place in the freezer for 20 minutes.

Servings: 4

Upgrade!
This recipe is a great replacement for **peanut butter cups** or any **candy bar.**

▶ POSTWORKOUT ▶ NUTRIENT-PACKED TREAT ▶ GLUTEN FREE ▶ DAIRY FREE ▶ VEGAN ▶ LOW FODMAP

PART II

Beverage Swaps

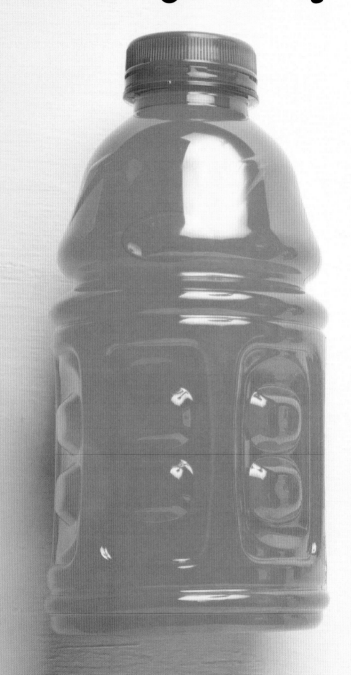

"Quench your thirst with food coloring ..."

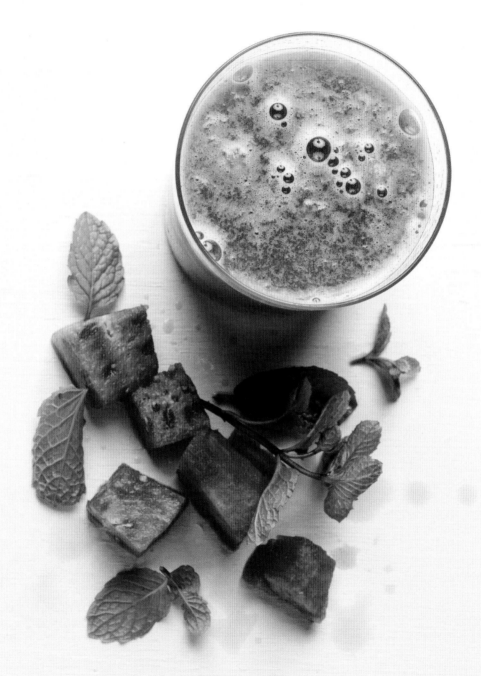

"or fuel your body?"

7

Sports Drinks, Energy Drinks, and Juices

Making juice from scratch allows you to drink your nutrients in the freshest way possible. Our recipes are mostly fruit and vegetable blends, but if you are trying to lose weight, always use more vegetables than fruit. If you enjoy having a glass of juice as part of a healthy morning routine, we recommend investing in a high-performance blender so you include fiber (the skins and seeds). Fiber found in nature's plants has many benefits. It slows down the release of sugar into the bloodstream and helps provide stable energy levels. Using a juicer is great, too. We try to keep the skins from the back of the juicer and add them to muffins. They're so tasty!

We recommend limiting commercial energy drinks and sports drinks because they contain some artificial and synthetic ingredients that may leave you more drained than energized. Try our natural drinks for real energy and natural hydration. No bogus claims and no crash afterward. It's worth the few extra minutes spent in the kitchen.

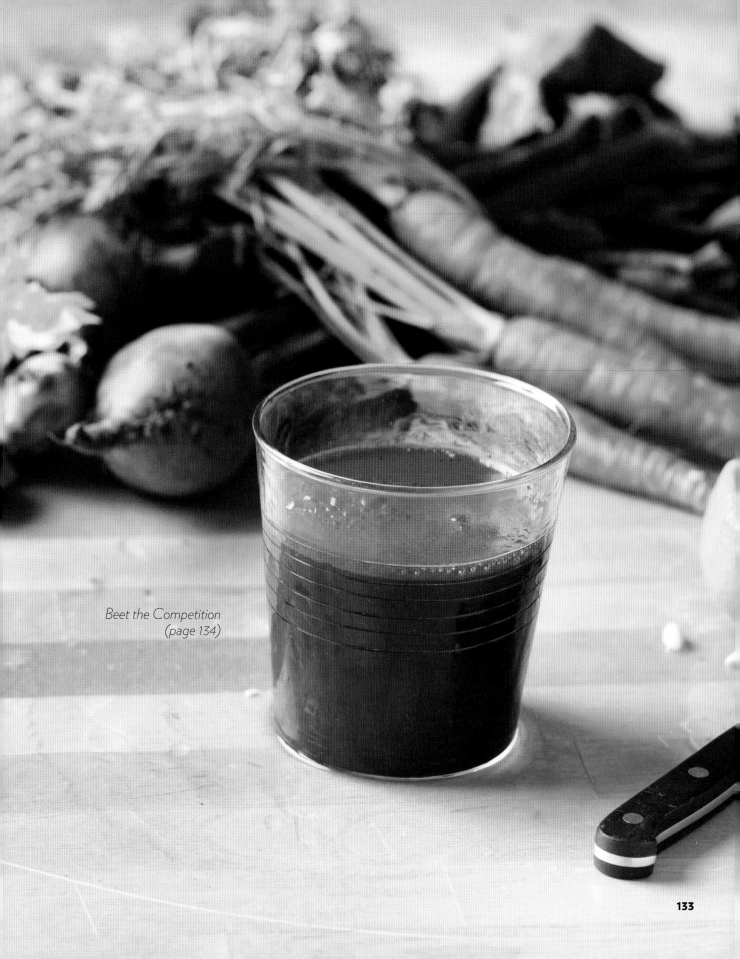

Beet the Competition
(page 134)

Beet the Competition

Beets are an endurance athlete's best friend because they have been shown to increase oxygen and blood flow to the muscles, helping to increase athletic performance. Sports-nutrition supplement companies have created powders and concentrated juice shot supplements to market to athletes. We think you get the greatest benefit from consuming beets fresh from the ground. Can't beet 'em.

1 medium beet
1 carrot
¼ lemon, peeled
2 celery stalks
2 teaspoons (4 g)
   fresh ginger, chopped

Juice all ingredients in a juicer, or place them in a high performance blender and blend until smooth.

Servings: 2

Notes: Add ½ cup (118 ml) water if using a blender.

Upgrade!
This recipe is a great replacement for **pasteurized beet juice** or **nitric oxide supplements.**

DID YOU KNOW? **Beets are naturally packed with nitrates. The body converts nitrates to nitric oxide, which helps with blood flow. Some elite athletes drink fresh beet juice before an intense workout or competition. About 2 cups (500 ml) is the ideal amount. Other good sources of nitrates are spinach, celery, radishes, lettuce, and Chinese cabbage. Cooking dampens some of the nitrates, so eating the vegetables raw is best.**

▶ PREWORKOUT ▶ POSTWORKOUT ▶ GLUTEN FREE ▶ DAIRY FREE ▶ VEGAN

Chocolate Raspberry Energy Shake

Supplement companies love marketing to athletes, who are always hungry for an extra boost. Some companies claim their energy shots are equal to consuming vegetables. Sorry, we're not buying it. The ingredients are synthetic, counterproductive, and can even block the absorption of electrolytes and nutrients. Try this shot when you need a real energy boost.

- 2 tablespoons (10 g) raw cacao powder
- 1 teaspoon green coffee bean powder or matcha powder
- 1 cup (235 ml) water
- ½ cup (75 g) frozen raspberries
- 3 drops ginseng
- 1 tablespoon (20 g) pure maple syrup

Combine all ingredients in a blender until smooth.

Servings: 2

Upgrade! This recipe is a great replacement for **energy shots** and **energy drinks**—and **coffee.**

DID YOU KNOW? Green coffee bean powder is made from unroasted young coffee beans, which have more antioxidants and more energy-providing nutrients than roasted coffee beans.

▶ PREWORKOUT ▶ NUTRIENT-PACKED TREAT ▶ GLUTEN FREE ▶ DAIRY FREE ▶ VEGAN

Lemon~Lime Quencher

It's important to drink liquids to hydrate, but most conventional sports drinks have food dyes, additives, and lots of sugar. Too much sugar can lead to gastrointestinal distress while training. Conventional sports nutrition wisdom says that sports drinks should have 6 to 8 percent sugar but some emerging research has shown that 4 to 5 percent is optimal.

- 3 cups (750 ml) water
- Juice and zest of 1 lemon
- Juice of 1 lime
- 2 teaspoons (40 g) pure maple syrup
- ¼ teaspoon Celtic sea salt or Himalayan pink sea salt

Combine all ingredients in a 24-ounce (710 ml) water bottle and shake vigorously.

Servings: 2

Notes: *To hydrate properly and avoid cramping, it is important to use a high-quality sea salt. Sea salt has trace minerals like potassium, magnesium, calcium, and chloride and electrolytes that your body needs to replenish itself.*

Upgrade! This recipe is a great replacement for **traditional sports drinks.**

▶ PREWORKOUT ▶ POSTWORKOUT ▶ GLUTEN FREE ▶ DAIRY FREE ▶ VEGAN ▶ LOW FODMAP

Anything but Sapped

Mother Nature is the best chemist and this nutrient-rich refresher taps into that natural power. Combining two incredible hydrators, this high-electrolyte drink helps prevent dehydration and fatigue. If you're feeling dehydrated, add a pinch of sea salt to replace excess sodium loss.

1 cup (154 g) of seedless watermelon

½ cup (160 g) maple water

½ cup (115 g) ice

6 leaves fresh mint

¼ teaspoon sea salt

Combine all ingredients in a blender and blend until smooth.

Servings: 2

Notes: *Kate and her triathlon training partner Jeff Rose are cofounders of DRINKmaple, a maple water company based in Concord, Massachusetts. Check out drinkmaple.com.*

DID YOU KNOW? Maple water is the sap that comes straight from maple trees. Traditionally, this sap is boiled down to make maple syrup. Maple sap has a waterlike consistency and is a natural hydration drink. It contains minerals, polyphenols, and antioxidants. The sugar is naturally created from the photosynthesis of the tree. Surprisingly, the sugar content is very low, about half the amount of sugar in coconut water.

❯ PREWORKOUT ❯ POSTWORKOUT ❯ GLUTEN FREE ❯ DAIRY FREE ❯ VEGAN

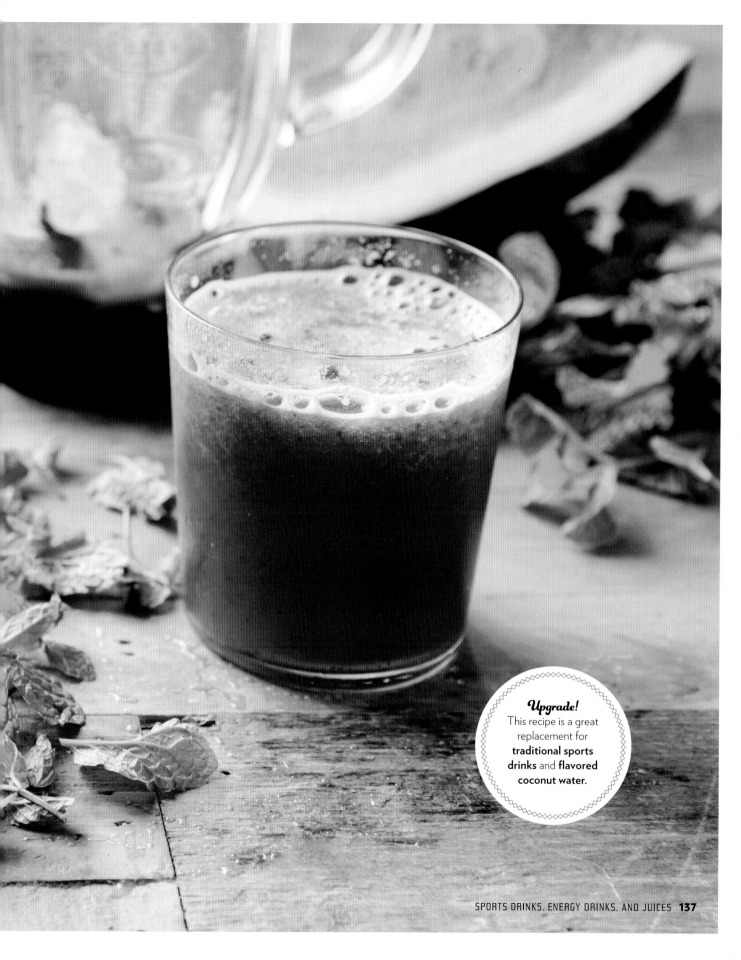

Upgrade!
This recipe is a great replacement for **traditional sports drinks** and **flavored coconut water.**

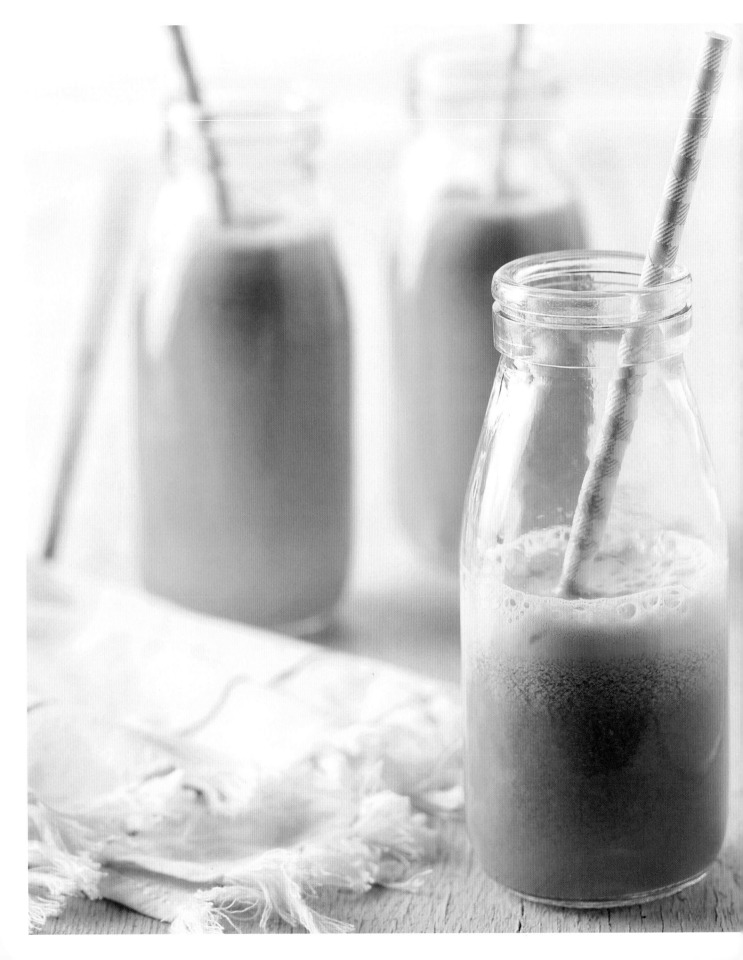

ACK Fresh Just Greens

We fell in love with this green juice from ACK Fresh on Nantucket Island because it is just greens without any fruit, making it lower in sugar than most juices. Green juices are packed with chlorophyll, which makes them great natural energizers. Try green juice in place of your energy drink for a pick me up. If you ever make a trip to Nantucket, stop by ACK Fresh and thank them for sharing this recipe or visit ackfresh.com.

1 cucumber

4 stalks celery

2 dandelion leaves

½ head of fennel

2 tablespoons (2 g) cilantro

½ lime, peeled

Juice all ingredients in a juicer or place them in a high-performance blender until smooth.

Servings: 2

Ugrade!
This recipe is a great replacement for **juice, coffee,** or **energy drinks.**

DID YOU KNOW? Dandelion greens aren't just the weeds that grow on your lawn; they are nutrient-rich greens. They have a bitter taste, so go easy on the amount you use until your taste adapts. A good source of iron, calcium, and vitamin C, dandelion greens are known for being a powerful detoxifier by stimulating the liver and helping to remove toxins.

"I'm probably the only person in the world that enjoys the taste of dandelions." —KATE

▶ PREWORKOUT ▶ POSTWORKOUT ▶ GLUTEN FREE ▶ DAIRY FREE ▶ VEGAN

Pucker Up Shots

You'll either love them or hate them. There's no middle ground here. But you may just warm up to our pickle juice and lemon shots when you find out how efficient they are as a pre-, during, or postworkout elixir for preventing muscle cramps. Who's in?

2 ounces (60 ml) pickle juice

Juice of 1 lemon

With your favorite 1-ounce (28 ml) shot glass, measure 2 shots of pickle juice and put them into a mason jar with a secure lid.

Add the lemon juice and shake well.

To serve, pour into 2 small glasses or shot glasses. Down the hatch!

Servings: 2 (or 1 serving for a "salty sweater")

Notes: Athletes who sweat a lot during exercise, also known as "salty sweaters," may suffer from muscle cramps due to dehydration and the loss of electrolytes. Pickle juice helps replenish the sodium efficiently. If it's not practical to drink a Pucker Up during a long event or race, try having a shot about 30 to 45 minutes before you start. The shots may help right after a long endurance event, too.

Upgrade!
This is a great replacement for **sports drinks** or **powdered electrolyte mixes**.

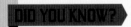 Not all pickles are created equal. Be sure to read the ingredient labels and look for varieties without added sugar, food dyes, or ingredients you can't pronounce.

▶ PREWORKOUT ▶ POSTWORKOUT ▶ GLUTEN FREE ▶ DAIRY FREE ▶ VEGAN

Sporty Spa Cubes

Water can be boring, but not drinking it makes it hard to keep up with hydration goals for optimal performance. These zesty ice cubes can be made with anything you have in the refrigerator that will add flavor. Fancy enough to dress up your water, but not so fancy that they require much effort.

1 ice cube tray (larger squares or fun shapes preferred)

1 cup (96 g) fresh mint, finely chopped

1 cucumber, coarsely chopped

1 lemon, zest first and then coarsely chopped

Water

Mix mint, cucumber, lemon, and lemon zest together.

Spoon equal amounts of the mixture into the ice cube squares. Add water slowly to fill trays. Freeze.

Servings: 4 to 6

Notes: *Some of our other favorite combinations are strawberries with mint, lime with basil and cucumber, and Meyer lemon with raspberries.*

Upgrade!
This recipe is a great replacement for **plain water** or **bottled flavored water.**

▶ PREWORKOUT ▶ POSTWORKOUT ▶ GLUTEN FREE ▶ DAIRY FREE ▶ VEGAN ▶ LOW FODMAP

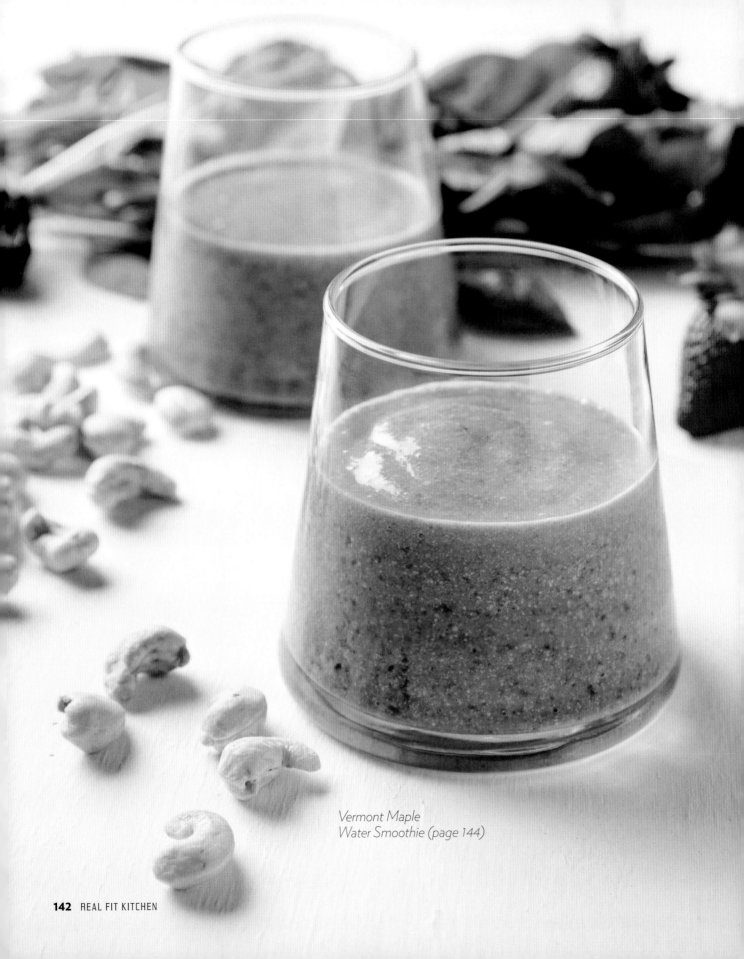

*Vermont Maple
Water Smoothie (page 144)*

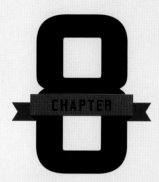

Smoothies and Milks

Smoothies should be simple. A great blender, a well-stocked kitchen, and about 2 minutes of time is all you need. Our protein smoothies and milks will feed your muscles with just a few natural ingredients that blend easily and taste delicious. It's really that simple. No lab coats, no chemicals.

Vermont Maple Water Smoothie

This recipe is great for anyone who is new to green smoothies. It is a great way to sneak some more greens into your diet by drinking what tastes like a strawberry milkshake.

1 cup (255 g) frozen strawberries
¼ cup (34 g) raw cashews
1 tablespoon (11 g) chia seeds
2 Medjool dates
½ teaspoon vanilla
½ cup (115 g) ice
½ cup (30 g) baby spinach
1 cup (250 ml) maple water

Combine all ingredients in a blender and blend until smooth.

Servings: 2

Upgrade!
This recipe is a great replacement for **milkshakes** or **protein shakes.**

DID YOU KNOW? **Strawberries are rich in vitamin C, which helps with iron absorption from plant-based foods. The strawberries and spinach are a tag team that work together to optimize the nutrition potential.**

▶ POST-WORKOUT ▶ GLUTEN FREE ▶ DAIRY FREE ▶ VEGAN

Cashew Chia Milk

Dairy-free milk is great for you, and making your own is surprisingly easy. To save time, you can make a batch at the beginning of the week and store it in mason jars in the refrigerator for up to a week.

1 cup (137 g) raw cashews
3½ cups (875 ml) water
1 tablespoon (11 g) chia seeds
1 Medjool dates or
2 tablespoons (40 g) pure maple syrup
½ teaspoon vanilla extract
¼ teaspoon sea salt

Combine all ingredients in a high-performance blender and blend until smooth. Adjust the number of dates or amount of maple syrup according to taste.

Servings: 2

Notes: You can substitute any nut for the cashews and choose which flavors you like best. See our note (page 146) about presoaking nuts and using a nut milk bag.

Upgrade!
This recipe is a great replacement for **milk** or **vanilla milkshakes.**

▶ POSTWORKOUT ▶ GLUTEN FREE ▶ DAIRY FREE ▶ VEGAN
*Low FODMAP–friendly: Use raw pepitas in place of the cashews and omit the dates.

Creamy Piña Colada Smoothie

Jenna, the founder of Green Blender, a smoothie delivery company, created this smoothie as an ode to the piña colada. She wanted to "up the nutritional ante" by adding a few embellishments such as cauliflower and spirulina. Cauliflower contains phytonutrients called *glucosinolates* that may help activate the body's detoxification system. When you blend cauliflower, it becomes creamy. Spirulina strengthens the immune system, improves digestion, and reduces inflammation.

When Jenna is not creating her latest blend, she is training for endurance events or writing about health and fitness. You can find out more at greenblender.com.

2 cups (60 g) spinach
½ cup (85 g) pineapple
1 banana
2 florets cauliflower
2 tablespoons (10 g) coconut flakes
1 teaspoon spirulina
1 cup (250 ml) water
1 cup ice

Combine all the ingredients in a blender until smooth.

Servings: 2

Upgrade!
This recipe is a great replacement for **supersweet, tropical fruit.**

DID YOU KNOW? Spirulina is a blue-green algae, one that boasts quite an impressive nutritional profile. An excellent source of B vitamins, vitamin C, vitamin D, and vitamin E, it is also high in potassium, chromium, copper, magnesium, manganese, phosphorus, selenium, sodium, and zinc. Studies show it may help to strengthen the immune system, improve digestion, and reduce inflammation. Algae is a great way to help your body bounce back after a workout.

▸ POSTWORKOUT ▸ GLUTEN FREE ▸ DAIRY FREE ▸ VEGAN

Chocolate Almond Milk

Chocolate milk is touted as the ideal recovery drink for athletes. While it is true that chocolate milk has a good mix of carbohydrates and protein to help your body recover, it has many other ingredients that can adversely affect your body. Our chocolate almond milk is loaded with nutrients and anti-inflammatory properties. Make it ahead of time so, at the end of your workout, you have something that will truly help you replenish.

1 cup (145 g) raw almonds

3½ cups (875 ml) water

1 teaspoon raw cacao powder

4 tablespoons (80 g) pure maple syrup

½ teaspoon vanilla extract

¼ teaspoon sea salt

⅛ teaspoon maca powder (optional)

Combine all ingredients in a blender and blend until smooth. Adjust the number of dates or amount of maple syrup according to your taste.

Servings: 2

Notes: *We like the consistency of this milk (and the quick recipe), but if you prefer a thinner milk you can strain it using a nut milk bag, which you can purchase online or at your local health food store.*

Upgrade!
This recipe is a great replacement for **chocolate milk** or **packaged recovery shakes or conventional/ almond milks.**

DID YOU KNOW? Soaking nuts may enhance the body's ability to digest the nutrients and will ensure blending a smoother milk. If you have the time, first soak the almonds in a bowl of cold water overnight (or for at least 5 hours). It will unlock the enzymes, allowing you to absorb more from this nutrient-rich food.

▶ POSTWORKOUT ▶ GLUTEN FREE ▶ DAIRY FREE ▶ VEGAN

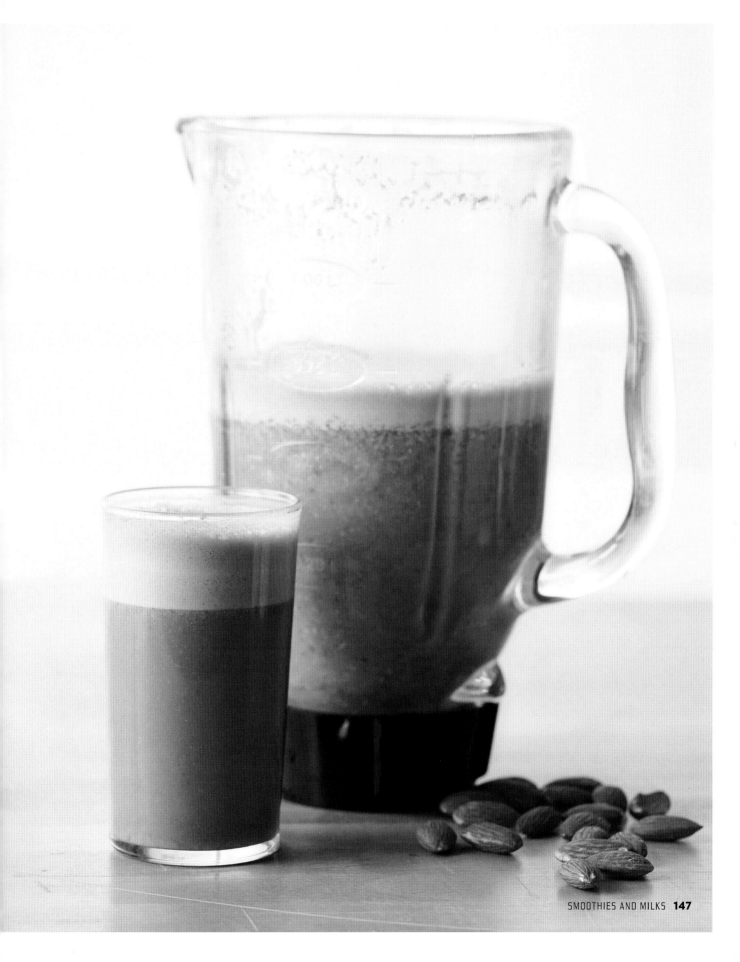

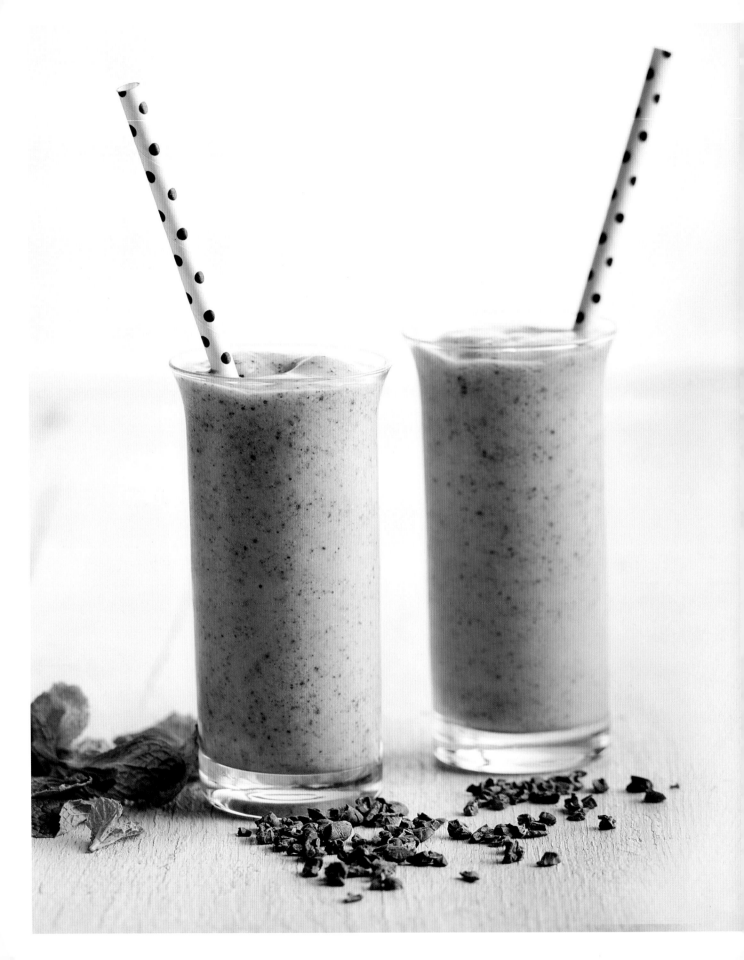

Mint Chip Smoothie

This smoothie has all the taste of our favorite childhood treat, a mint chocolate chip ice cream cone, but packs in a whole heck of a lot more nutrition!

1½ (375 ml) cups maple water (or plain water)

¼ cup (38 g) raw almonds

1 cup (30 g) spinach

12 fresh mint leaves

1 frozen banana

½ avocado

1 tablespoon (11 g) raw cacao nibs

1 teaspoon vanilla

2 tablespoons (40 g) pure maple syrup

1 cup ice

Combine all the ingredients in a high-speed blender until smooth.

Servings: 2

Notes: *Be adventurous and switch up the spinach with other greens like kale, swiss chard, or collard greens. Keep in mind that of these greens, spinach has the mildest flavor.*

Ugrade!
This recipe is a great replacement for **milkshakes** or **conventional smoothies.**

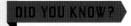 **Mint has been used for hundreds of years for its medicinal properties. It promotes digestion by calming and soothing an upset stomach or indigestion.**

▶ POSTWORKOUT ▶ NUTRIENT-PACKED TREAT ▶ GLUTEN FREE ▶ DAIRY FREE
▶ VEGAN ▶ LOW FODMAP

Get Buzzed Smoothie

This smoothie gives you the extra energy you need with its caffeine, maca, and chia, but without the predictable crash you get from popular coffee drinks that taste great but are loaded with sugar.

- 1 cup (250 ml) cold brew liquid coffee concentrate (unsweetened)
- 1 cup (250 ml) maple water (or plain water)
- 1 teaspoon maca powder
- 2 tablespoons (22 g) chia seeds
- 2 tablespoons (40 g) pure maple syrup
- ¼ cup (34 g) raw cashews
- 1 teaspoon vanilla
- 1 cup (230 g) ice

Combine all ingredients in a high-speed blender and enjoy.

Servings: 2

Upgrade!
This recipe is a great replacement for **milkshakes, lattes, frappes, coffee drinks,** or **conventional smoothies.**

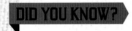 **DID YOU KNOW?**   Cold brewed coffee liquid is less acidic—so it's easier on the stomach and better for bone health.

▶ POSTWORKOUT ▶ NUTRIENT-PACKED TREAT ▶ GLUTEN FREE ▶ DAIRY FREE ▶ VEGAN
* Low FODMAP-friendly: Use raw almonds in place of the cashews.

Spicy Chocolate Volcano Smoothie

This spicy smoothie is a creamy, drinkable version of a decadent molten chocolate dessert. Jenna at Green Blender swapped out the sugar and butter for fiber and potassium.

2 cups (60 g) spinach
1 banana
½ avocado
1 tablespoon (5 g) raw cacao powder
1 teaspoon cinnamon
⅛ teaspoon cayenne pepper
1 cup (250 ml) water
½ cup (115 g) ice

Combine all the ingredients in a blender until smooth.

Servings: 2

Upgrade!
This recipe is a great replacement for **milkshakes** and **packaged recovery drinks.**

▶ POSTWORKOUT ▶ GLUTEN FREE ▶ DAIRY FREE ▶ VEGAN ▶ LOW FODMAP

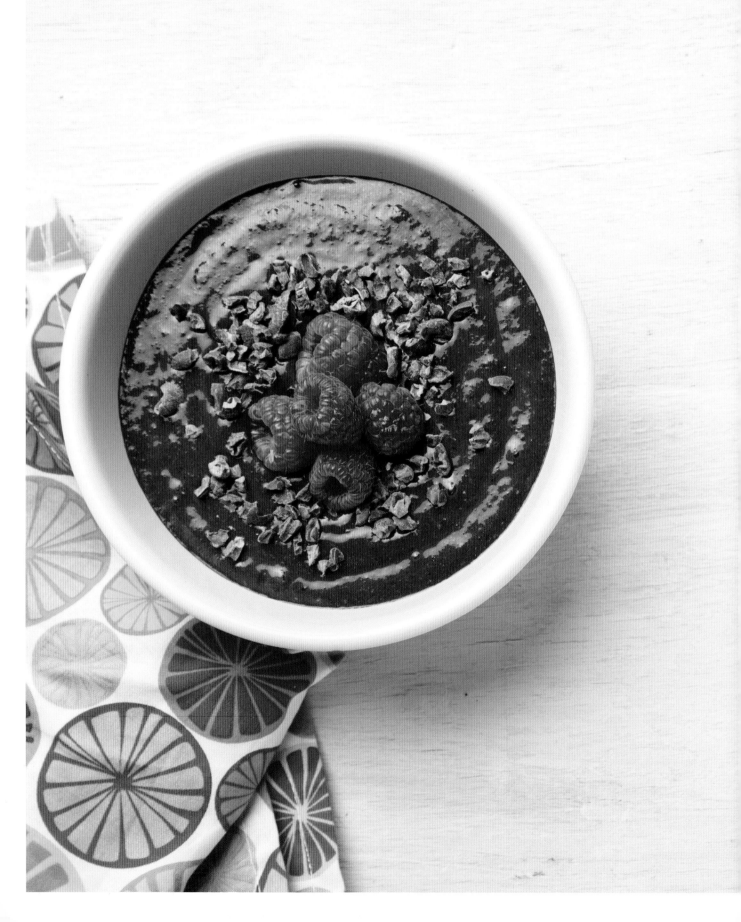

Chocolate Recovery Pudding

This pudding is a recovery smoothie in a bowl. It is Kate's go-to breakfast on Iron-man training days. People always ask for the recipe after seeing her eat this at work meetings or training sessions.

- 2 cups (310 g) frozen cherries
- 1 cup (67 g) kale or spinach, stems removed
- 2 tablespoons (11 g) raw cacao powder

- 1½ tablespoons (16 g) chia seeds
- 1 tablespoon (9 g) natural protein powder (hemp or sprouted brown rice protein)
- ½ teaspoon maca powder

- 1 tablespoon (11 g) cacao nibs
- 1 tablespoon (12 g) grass-fed gelatin (optional)
- 2 dates, raw honey or pure maple syrup to taste (optional)

Combine all the ingredients except the cacao nibs in a high-performance blender or food processor and blend until smooth.

To serve, top with cacao nibs and fresh fruit such as figs, bananas, berries, or pomegranates.

Servings: 2

Notes: *For a milder taste, use baby kale or baby spinach. If your blender has a plunger, use that to help with the blending. If it's too thick, slowly add a bit of water to thin it out.*

▶ POSTWORKOUT ▶ NUTRIENT-PACKED TREAT ▶ GLUTEN FREE ▶ DAIRY FREE ▶ VEGAN

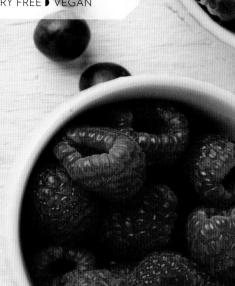

III

Supplement and Pill Swaps

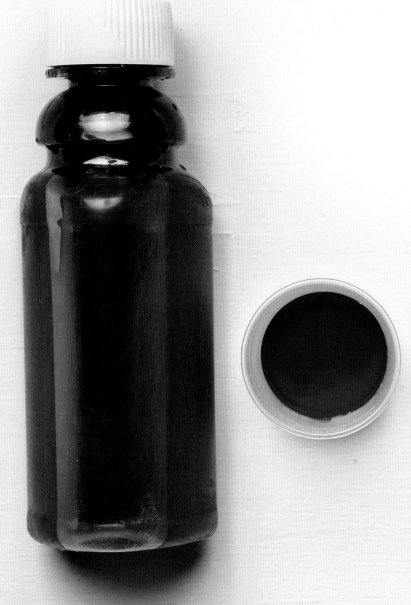

"From over the counter ..."

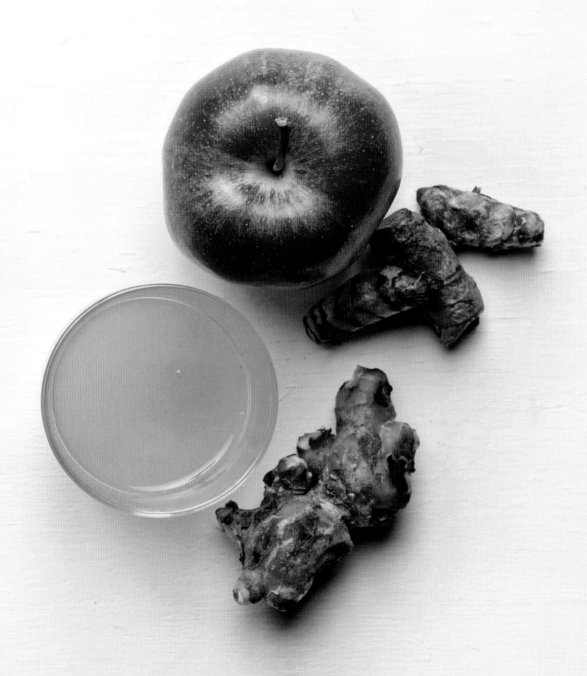

"to fresh from the farm."

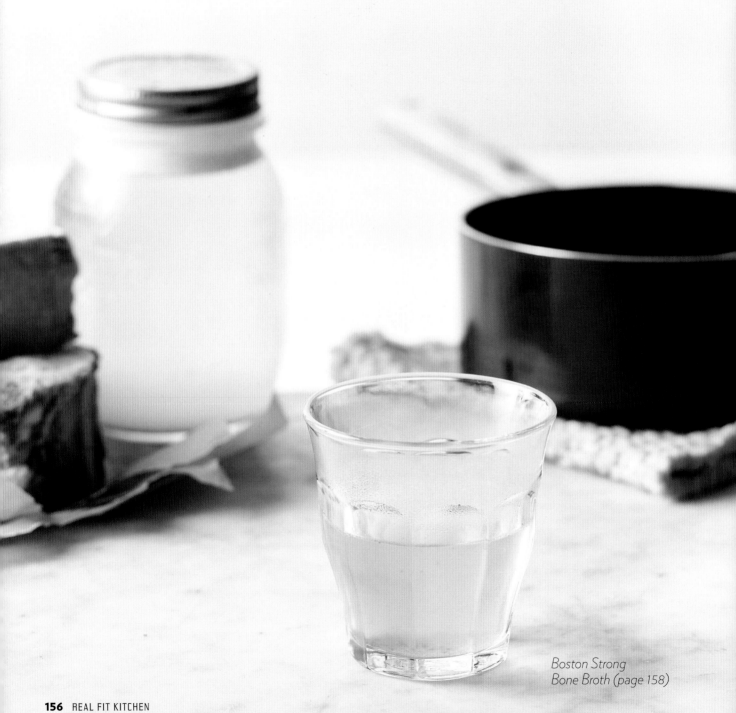

Boston Strong
Bone Broth (page 158)

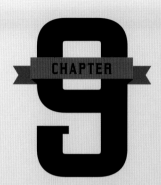

CHAPTER 9

Anti~Inflammatory Solutions

The stress of modern life inevitably results in inflammation in the body. Inflammation is part of the body's immune response, which helps us heal by attacking and destroying bacteria and viruses. When it's out of control, however, inflammation can cause problems in the heart, joints, mood, and even in memory. Some stressors can push the inflammatory response too far, such as excessive exercise, lack of sleep, too much stress, and poor food choices.

Because both acute and chronic inflammation are a part of everyday life, it makes sense to do whatever possible to decrease them. There are detox formulas, antioxidants, essential fatty acids, joint support, and memory enhancers, all available as pills or powders.

Instead of those over-the-counter aids, we advocate getting as many anti-inflammatories from real food as you can. Mindful eating, slowing down, regular relaxation, and laughter can enhance your overall strategy.

Boston Strong Bone Broth

Aloe-ha Vera Shots

Fire Cider Shots

Turmeric Tonic Shot

Creamy Turmeric Latte

Minty Nettle Elixir

Killer Sauerkraut

Healing Gummy Snacks

Easy Injera

Boston Strong Bone Broth

This recipe may seem intimidating at first (bones, and 24 hours to cook, really?), but it is surprisingly easy to make with a little organization. We have experienced the benefits of bone broth ourselves and some of our athletes swear by it.

8	cups (2 L) water
2 to 3	leg bones from a grass-fed cow
3	carrots, coarsely chopped
4	celery stalks, roughly chopped
1	onion, peeled and coarsely chopped
2	garlic cloves, peeled and coarsely chopped
3	tablespoons (44 ml) unfiltered apple cider vinegar
	Juice of 1 lemon
1	teaspoon sea salt

Preheat the oven to 350°F (180°C).

Put the bones on a baking sheet and roast for 20 minutes.

Fill a large soup pot with the water, add the remaining ingredients along with the bones, and bring to a rolling boil.

Reduce the heat to very low and simmer covered for 24 to 48 hours.

Strain out the bones, carrots, celery, onion and garlic out and pour the broth into mason jars.

Refrigerate the jars and heat a portion when you are ready to drink.

For best results, drink the broth on an empty stomach or after a workout.

Servings: 8 to 10

Notes: For this recipe, you want bones from the legs of the cow. You can find grass-fed bones from local farms or at a natural grocery store. This recipe is also perfect for a slow cooker.

Upgrade!
This recipe is a great replacement for **glucosomine, chondroitin,** or **glutamine supplements, pills,** or **powders.**

DID YOU KNOW? Bone broth naturally contains glucosomine, chondroitin, and hyaluronic acid, all of which are beneficial to joint health and general gastrointestinal health. With a strong gastrointestinal system, you can digest food more efficiently and absorb more nutrients. What great reasons to make bone broth part of your routine!

▶ POSTWORKOUT ▶ GLUTEN FREE ▶ DAIRY FREE
*Low FODMAP–friendly: Omit garlic and onions.

Aloe~ha Vera Shots

Taking aloe shots after tough training sessions became a ritual for Kate when she was training for an Ironman. These shots are not delicious, but they are a top recovery strategy because they are a powerful anti-inflammatory. Aloe also helps soothe the digestive system. This natural strategy works to lessen and prevent pain.

1 aloe vera leaf
3 cups (750 ml) water
   (or fresh orange juice)

Cut off the ends of the aloe leaf, slit the leaf down the middle, and remove the aloe fillet (inner gel) with a spoon.

Put the aloe gel in a blender with the water or juice and blend for 2 minutes.

Put the mixture in a jar and keep it in the refrigerator.

Take one 4-ounce (30 ml) shot daily or after tough training sessions.

Servings: 6

Notes: *If making your own aloe shot is not something that appeals to you, look for a commercial aloe juice that is free of preservatives, sugar, or other additives. Find a brand that has one ingredient: pure aloe juice.*

Upgrade!
To us, this is a great replacement for **NSAIDs** such as **ibuprofen.** When we have aloe on hand, this is our go-to for lessening the burn.

DID YOU KNOW? Aloe is one of the oldest known medicinal plants and was called the "plant of immortality" by the Egyptians. It has anti-inflammatory properties and may help reduce the pain and stiffness from arthritis and ease muscle and joint pain. You can find aloe leaves at natural health food stores and at tropical markets.

▶ POSTWORKOUT ▶ GLUTEN FREE ▶ DAIRY FREE ▶ VEGAN

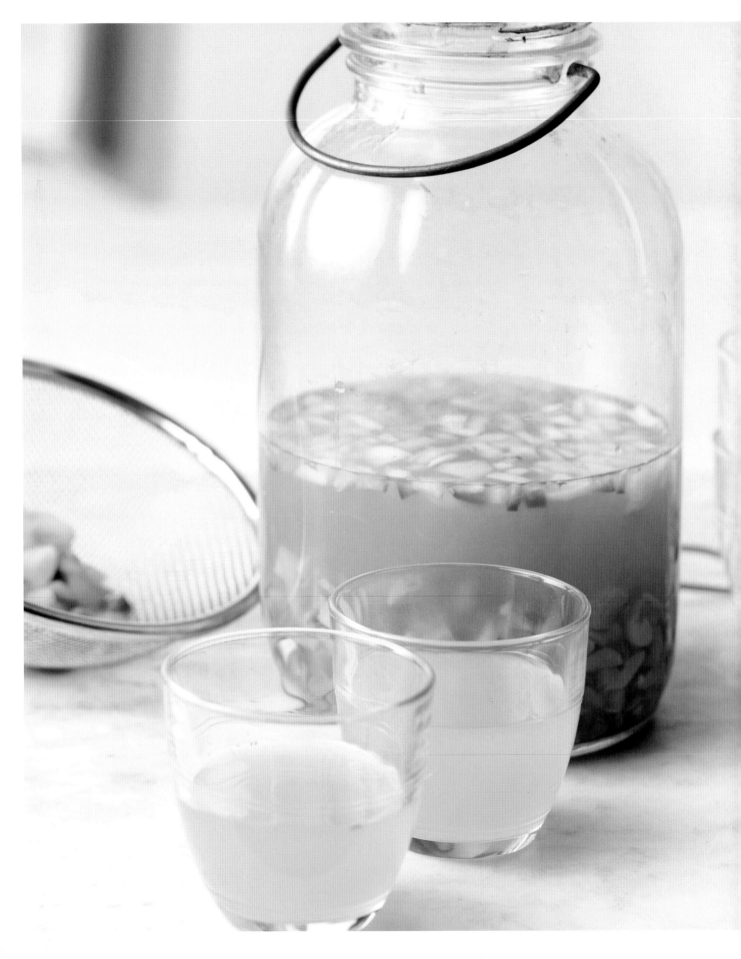

Fire Cider Shots

Fire cider is an old folk remedy that has been consumed for hundreds of years. The combination of the powerful antibacterial, anti-inflammatory, and antimicrobial properties helps you fight off colds, improve digestion, and boost your immune system naturally. Some athletes drink a preventive shot every morning, especially during cold and flu season. (This isn't the best-tasting shot, but it will likely help you keep you healthy and strong.)

- 3 cups (750 ml) raw unfiltered apple cider vinegar
- ½ cup garlic, peeled and chopped
- ½ cup (80 g) onion, peeled and chopped
- ½ cup (50 g) fresh horseradish root, chopped
- ½ cup (50 g) turmeric root, chopped
- ¼ cup (50 g) organic ginger root, chopped
- 1 habanero or jalapeño chile, chopped
- ½ organic orange or grapefruit, chopped
- ½ organic lemon, chopped
- 1 tablespoon (20 g) raw honey, or to taste (optional)

Combine all the ingredients in a large mason jar and cover securely.

Let the jar sit at room temerature for 3 to 4 weeks, giving it a shake every couple of days.

Strain the mixture and pour it into a fresh jar.

Refrigerate and take a shot daily.

Servings: 12

Notes: *Make this before cold season starts so you have it when everyone around you begins to get sick. If you prefer, you can purchase good-quality fire cider at a natural health food store or online. As always, check the ingredients list. We make a big batch and keep it in the refrigerator during the winter months.*

Upgrade!
This recipe is a great replacement for **cold medicine** or a **decongestant.**

DID YOU KNOW? While there is time and place for medication (always listen to your doctor), we encourage you to try this traditional remedy for preventing a cold. Many over-the-counter cold medicines have artificial ingredients and food dyes.

▶ GLUTEN FREE ▶ DAIRY FREE
*Vegan: Use pure maple syrup instead of honey.

Turmeric Tonic Shot

Turmeric has been used for years in India as a powerful healing root. We saw our athletes move a little easier and feel more energized after incorporating turmeric into their foods and smoothies. If you are feeling adventurous, you can take a shot of this spicy tonic straight up. If you like it a little sweeter, add some raw honey or pure maple syrup to make it more palatable for your taste.

1 piece fresh turmeric root, about 4-inches (10 cm) long (or 2 teaspoons [4.4 g] turmeric)

1 piece fresh ginger root, about 4-inches long

4 cups (1 L) water

pinch black pepper

Raw honey to taste

Combine all the ingredients in a high-performance blender for 2 minutes.

Consume immediately or pour the mixture into a mason jar and refrigerate.

Servings: 8

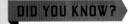 **DID YOU KNOW?** Studies have shown that black pepper increases the body's absorption of turmeric when the two are consumed together.

▶ PREWORKOUT ▶ POSTWORKOUT ▶ GLUTEN FREE ▶ DAIRY FREE
*Vegan: Use pure maple syrup instead of honey.

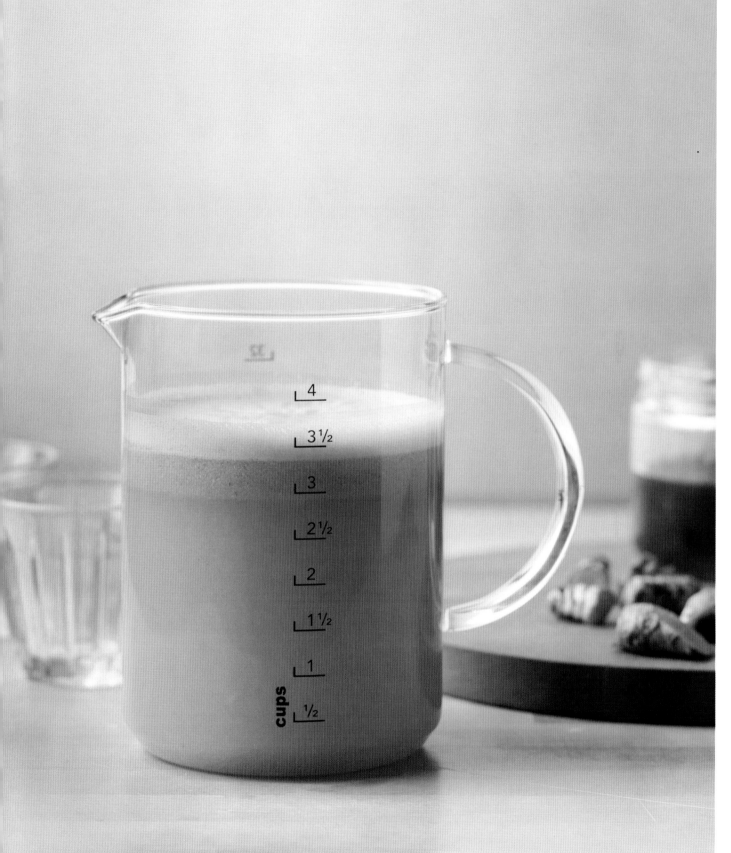

Creamy Turmeric Latte

One of our top recovery tips is to incorporate more turmeric root. The question is always about how to eat it without eating curry every night. We asked Elise of Kale and Chocolate to give us her favorite turmeric recipe, and she created this delicious latte that can be enjoyed any time of day. For more about Elise and her recipes, visit her website at kaleandchocolate.com.

1 cup (250 ml) unsweet-ened almond milk

1 heaping tablespoon (6 g) fresh turmeric root, grated (or 2 teaspoons turmeric paste, see notes)

1 tablespoon (6 g) fresh gingerroot, grated (or 1 teaspoon ground ginger)

1 teaspoon cinnamon

1 tablespoon (14 g) coconut oil or ghee

Pure maple syrup to taste

Gently warm the almond or coconut milk in a small saucepan, but do not bring it to a boil. Add the turmeric, ginger, and cinnamon.

Add the coconut oil to the milk mixture and heat until it is melted.

Stir in honey to taste.

Use a wire whisk or immersion blender to create foam, if you like.

Servings: 1

Notes: *If you can't find fresh turmeric root, make turmeric paste by mixing 2 teaspoons (4.4 g) ground turmeric with 2 teaspoons (10 ml) water.*

❯ NUTRIENT-PACKED TREAT ❯ GLUTEN FREE ❯ DAIRY FREE ❯ VEGAN ❯ LOW FODMAP

Minty Nettle Elixir

Kate's massage therapist introduced us to nettle tea. She raved about the powerful benefits of stinging nettle and how it has helped so many of her athletes reduce the symptoms of allergies, exercise-induced asthma, and reduced overall fatigue.

¼ cup (115 g) dried nettle

½ cup (192 g) fresh mint, or dried

4 cups (1 L) water

Put the nettles and water in a small saucepan and bring to a boil.

Reduce to low heat and let simmer for 5 minutes.

Strain nettle and mint leaves.

Enjoy hot or store it in mason jars in the refrigerator for a cold tea elixir.

Servings: 4

Notes: You can find dried nettle at your local health food store or online at avenabotanicals.com. Even easier, you can purchase nettle tea bags in a natural grocery store.

DID YOU KNOW? Nettles have a long history, Shakespeare mentioned them in one of his plays. Nettles are high in iron, helping to generate new red blood cells and reduce fatigue, and a good source of calcium (430 grams of calcium in 1 cup).

▶ PREWORKOUT ▶ POSTWORKOUT ▶ GLUTEN FREE ▶ DAIRY FREE ▶ VEGAN ▶ LOW FODMAP

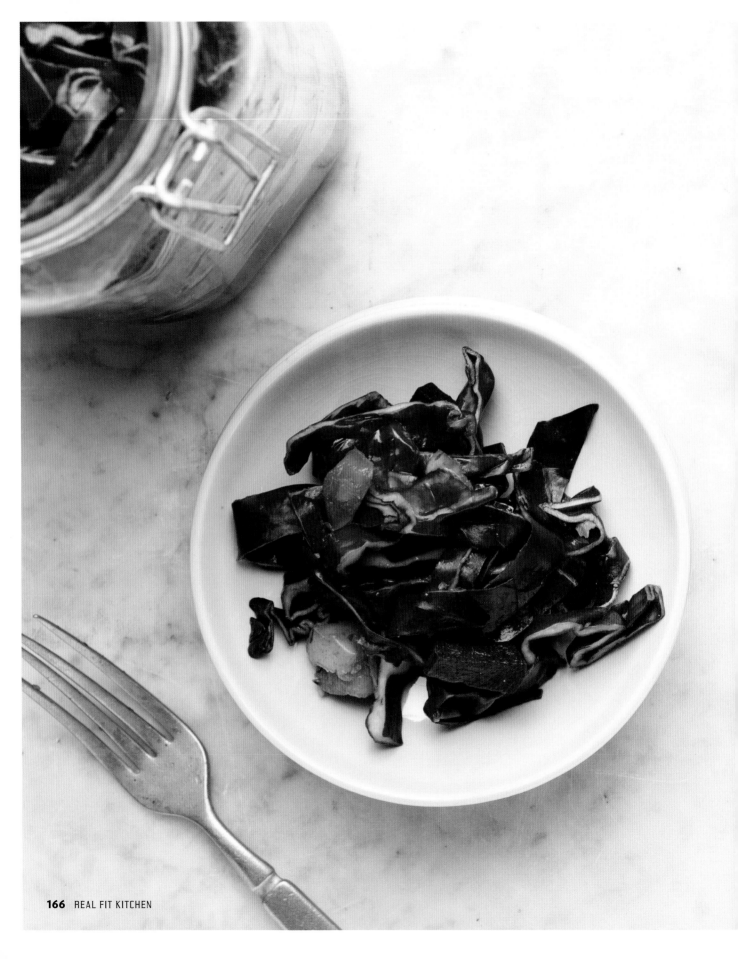

Killer Sauerkraut

Fermenting has been used for years as a method of preserving vegetables and the most common one is fermented cabbage or sauerkraut. When a vegetable is fermented in the traditional lacto-fermented way, it contains good probiotics that help boost intestinal health, improving the digestive tract and the absorption of nutrients. Eating fermented foods boosts your immune system, too. This recipe is easy to make, but requires some quality time to properly ferment.

1 head red or green cabbage, chopped

4 red beets, chopped

1 pear, chopped

1 teaspoon fresh ginger, chopped

1 tablespoon (18 g) sea salt

Combine all the ingredients in a bowl and use your hands to massage in the sea salt.

Place all ingredients in a sauerkraut crock, a large mason jar, or vegetable fermenter, making sure the ingredients are tightly packed.

If you are using a sauerkraut crock, place a weight on the sauerkraut to keep it packed. If you are using a mason jar, place a small jelly jar inside with a rock in it to keep it packed down and seal the jar tightly.

Let it sit in a cold, dry place for 1 to 2 months.

Remove the sauerkraut and place it in a clean jar in the refridgerator. It keeps for about 6 months.

Servings: 24

Notes: *When you buy sauerkraut, make sure you choose a brand with live probiotics. Good indicators that the sauerkraut is lacto-fermented: It doesn't have vinegar in the ingredients and it is in the refrigerated section of the store.*

Ugrade!
This recipe is a great replacement for **probiotic supplements.**

▶ POSTWORKOUT ▶ GLUTEN FREE ▶ DAIRY FREE ▶ VEGAN
*Low FODMAP–friendly: Omit the pear and use grapes instead.

Healing Gummy Snacks

These little snacks remind us of those childhood favorites but without the sugar rush. These gummy snacks are made with grass-fed gelatin, which may help with digestive health.

- 4 tablespoons (48 g) unflavored, grass-fed gelatin
- 1 cup (145 g) strawberries or mixed berries
- Juice of 1 lemon
- ⅓ cup (80 ml) water
- Pure maple syrup to taste (optional)

Blend together the lemon juice, strawberries, and water.

Put the mixture into a saucepan and heat on medium. Slowly mix in the gelatin and maple syrup and stir until the gelatin is dissolved.

Pour the mixture into candy molds, ice cube trays, or a small glass baking pan and refrigerate for 45 minutes.

If you used a pan, cut into small squares or use cookie cutters to make shapes.

Servings: 6

Notes: *You can make this like Jell-O by pouring the mixture into small bowls and refrigerating it. You can make different flavors by substituting other fruit like oranges, blueberries, cherries, or raspberries for the strawberries.*

Upgrade!
This recipe is a great replacement for **glucosamine** and **chondroitin supplements.**

▶ PREWORKOUT ▶ POSTWORKOUT ▶ GLUTEN FREE ▶ DAIRY FREE ▶ LOW FODMAP

Easy Injera

Injera is a traditional Ethiopian and Eritrean staple that is similar to a spongy, sourdough pancake. It is made with *teff*, a North African grass, rich in iron, fermented for a few days and is a great source of probiotics. Debra from Debra's Natural Gourmet, one of our favorite Boston-area natural health food stores, shared her recipe. Find more healthful tips at debrasnaturalgourmet.com.

1½ cups (198 g) teff flour

2 cups (500 ml) water

1 teaspoon sea salt

1 tablespoon (14 g) ghee, coconut oil, or (15 ml) extra-virgin olive oil

Mix the teff flour with the water and salt until the dough is smooth, without any lumps.

Let the dough stand in a bowl at room temperature, covered with a dish towel, until the mixture bubbles. This is will take 2 to 3 days.

Put the ghee or oil into a large skillet on medium heat.

Use a ¼-cup (60 ml) measuring cup to scoop the batter into the skillet. Cook each injera until bubbles form in the dough and the edges lift up from the pan. The bread will look like a pancake-like flatbread.

Let the injera cool. Place foil, wax paper, or paper towels between each piece, to prevent sticking.

Tear off pieces to eat plain or to scoop up dips or stews.

Servings: 4

Note: If you want the flatbread to be crispy and more like a chip, you can flip it to the other side and cook it for another minute.

Upgrade!
This recipe is an upgrade for **bread, flatbread, crackers,** and **chips.**

DID YOU KNOW? Teff can be used for more than making injera—as porridge to eat in the morning or serve it as a side dish. Teff is a great gluten-free grain that is rich in calcium, iron, fiber, and protein. Look for it in the grain aisle or at an African food–specialty store.

▶ PREWORKOUT ▶ POSTWORKOUT ▶ GLUTEN FREE ▶ DAIRY FREE ▶ LOW FODMAP

Acknowledgments

We both thank Jess Haberman, our Fair Winds Press acquiring editor. This project started with her from day one. She believed in us and coached us through the entire process. We also thank Betsy Gammons and Anne Re of Fair Winds for keeping us on track. Thanks to Kristin Teig and Catrine Kelty for making our recipes jump off the page with your gorgeous styling and photography. You two inspire us to get in the kitchen and play. We know your work will inspire our readers to do the same. Thanks to the various people who contributed recipes, allowing us to share your creativity with our readers. Thanks to Lisa Tener, our book writing coach. You're the one that made us DO THIS. Brainstorming the book concept seaside in Narragansett certainly helped the process.

Tara also thanks:
Kate: Thank you for DaBook. WE DID THIS! To Trish Leavitt of silverlining-design.com for your beautiful design work and genuine friendship: Your visual translation of my nutrition messages has changed my practice and helped so many of my clients, patients, and athletes along the way. The entire staff at Lown Cardiovascular Center and Dr. Jane Sillman of Brigham and Women's Hospital for believing that food can help, prevent, and heal. Dr. Dara Lee Lewis: for always keeping dark chocolate in her office. The dietitians at Dana-Farber Cancer Institute: I owe you for opening my eyes to the art of integrative nutrition. You elevated my game. Thanks also to: Mat Schaffer, Rebecca Pacheco, Dan Fitzgerald, Sally Sampson, Sandra Fairbank, Shannon Allen, Chef Todd Kiley, Daisy Chow, Kevin Kearns, November Project Boston, Brogan Graham, Bojan Mandaric, Nike+ Run Club Boston, Byron Ricketts, Mitchell Green, Jenn and Ben O'Meara, Chris "CanofSpaghetti" Cantergiani, Kosta, Barry Gagne, Ron Lawner, Lloyd Poindexter, and Wally's Cafe Jazz Club. Special thanks to Alicia Anskis and Gatsby for being so amazing, selfless, and reliable. Thanks to my nephews, Trent and Bryce. Stacey and Jon, you have the best kids in the world. Thanks to my parents, George and Bev: I love you. Your support is impossible to capture. I'm blessed. Lastly, to H. Eaton: Thank you for our daily conversations—a wink and a nod from heaven. It's all I need.

Kate also thanks:
Thank you to Tara for being an incredible partner on this journey and making this dream to write a book a reality. I am forever grateful that you responded to my email years ago and little did I know that the mentorship would lead to a great friendship and a published book. To my Mom and Dad for their love and overwhelming support in everything that I do: Thank you for instilling in me a sense of dedication and ambition and raising me to believe that I can do anything that I set my mind to. To my brother Michael and sister Meghan for their love and support. To my business partner, Jeff, who was beyond patient throughout this book-writing process as we were experiencing the craziness of start-up company life. Thank you for giving me a much-needed reality check every once in a while. To my clients who continually impress me with their dedication and tenacity. To all of my training partners and team members with whom I swim, bike, and run: Thank you for inspiring me, supporting me, and making me realize that this sport is more about being part of an incredible community than anything else.

About the Authors

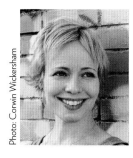

Photo: Corwin Wickersham

Tara Mardigan, M.S., M.P.H., R.D. is a Boston-based nutritionist, also known as The Plate Coach. She counsels clients and athletes at Lown Cardiovascular Center in Brookline, Massachusetts. She also consults in private practice and with the telemedicine company, FruitStreet.com. She is the head nutritionist for grown—real food, cooked slow for fast people—a restaurant concept sprouting in Miami. Her mission is to inspire others to find the most nourishing foods and lifestyle choices to meet their health needs and palates. She is a firm believer that, "Good for you should taste good, too."

Tara is the former team nutritionist for the Boston Red Sox. She helped the organization incorporate a food-first approach to optimize performance and win three World Series championships. She also worked with cancer survivors and their families at Dana-Farber Cancer Institute/Brigham and Women's Hospital for a decade.

Tara serves on the Food Task Force at Boston's Museum of Science to leverage food as an educational priority through the lenses of health sustainability, as well as the science, technology, and art of cooking. She is on the medical advisory boards for LighterCulture.com and Sjögren's Syndrome Foundation. She volunteers as the nutritionist for Team Sjögren's, the charity running team to raise awareness for Sjogren's Sydrome, a chronic autoimmune disease in which the body's moisture-producing glands are attacked.

Tara is a passionate member of Hubway, Boston's bike-share system and November Project, a free fitness movement formed in Boston. She has completed four Boston Marathons, several half marathons, and loves yoga, cycling, jazz, farm-to-table dinners, and the Adirondack Mountains.

Tara has a B.A. in nutrition science from the University of New Hampshire and completed her dietetic internship at Yale–New Haven Hospital. She holds M.S. and M.P.H. degrees from Tufts University.

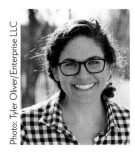

Photo: Tyler Oliver/Enterprise LLC

Kate Weiler, M.S., C.H.C., is a sports nutritionist who works with athletes to optimize athletic performance through nutrition. She has combined her strongly holistic mentality with the reality of what actually works and what is convenient for a time-pressed, busy athlete. Kate is also the co-founder and C.E.O. of DRINKmaple, which is a maple water beverage company.

Kate is an age-group elite triathlete who has completed five full-distance Ironman races, a countless number of triathlons, and more than ten marathons. She is a multiple-time qualifier and finisher of the Boston Marathon and is also qualifier and finisher of the Ironman World Championships in Kona, Hawaii.

Kate has a M.S. in nutrition from Northeastern University and earned her C.H.C. coaching certification from the Institute for Integrative Nutrition in New York. She has a Certificate of Integrative Nutrition from Purchase College, SUNY, and is certified by the American Association of Drugless Practitioners. She holds a B.A. from Colby College.

Index